Pain Relief for Life

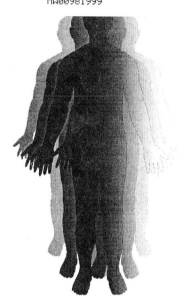

By

Al Skrobisch, C.N.M.T.

NEW PAGE BOOKS
A division of The Career Press, Inc.
Franklin Lakes, NJ

PAIN RELIEF FOR LIFE
EDITED BY JODI BRANDON
TYPESET BY EILEEN DOW MUNSON
Illustrations by Albert Chacon, Chacon Graphics
Cover design by Mada Design, Inc. / NYC
Printed in the U S A by Book-mart Press

To order this title, please call toll-free 1-800-CAREER-1 (NJ and Canada: 201-848-0310) to order using VISA or MasterCard, or for further information on books from Career Press.

The Career Press, Inc., 3 Tice Road, PO Box 687, Franklin Lakes, NJ 07417
www.careerpress.com
www.newpagebooks.com

This book is not intended to provide medical advice or to diagnose or treat any medical condition. The exercises, stretches, ideas, and recommendations presented are those the author has found helpful and effective in restoring proper muscular balance, creating good postural alignment, and reducing or eliminating pain. However, while they are time tested, based on common sense and sound principles, and have worked for many people, they may not be appropriate for you or your particular condition. Accordingly, it is recommended that you obtain the approval of your physician or other primary healthcare provider before beginning any exercise or stretching program. Also, there are other causes of pain, such as injury and disease, that are not within the scope of this book and may require other forms of treatment. These conditions should be ruled out by your physician or other primary healthcare provider before you begin this program.

The author and publisher specifically disclaim any responsibility for any liability, loss, or risk, whether personal or otherwise, which someone may incur as a consequence, directly or indirectly, of the use and application of any of the contents of this book.

Library of Congress Cataloging-in-Publication Data

Skrobisch, Al.
   Pain relief for life / by Al Skrobisch.
     p. cm.
   Includes bibliographical references and index.
   ISBN 1-56414-655-3 (pbk.)
    1. Pain—Treatment—Popular works. 2. Posture disorders—Therapy—Popular works. I. Title.

RB127.S55 2003
616'.0472—dc21

2002045247

*To Those Who form
a Guardian Wall
around suffering humanity,
selflessly serving, protecting, guiding,
and loving all that lives
because, for Them,
"there is no other Path at all to go,"
this book is humbly and gratefully dedicated.*

G. D. E. M. R.

Acknowledgments

I owe a sincere debt of gratitude to so many who have helped, in one way or another, to make this book possible. In particular, I want to express my appreciation to my agent, Pat Snell, for being willing to take a chance on representing a first-time author; to all the staff at New Page Books, for making the process so much easier and more comfortable than I expected; to Albert Chacon of Chacon Graphics, for his excellent illustrations and his patience with my desire to get them "just right"; to Janet Travell, M.D. and David G. Simons, M.D., for their definitive and fascinating two-volume work on Myofascial Pain and Dysfunction; to Paul St. John, L.M.T., for his dedication to researching and developing St. John Neuromuscular Therapy and making it such a powerful and effective healing modality; to all my clients and students, whose search for a way to end their pain or the pain of others has taught me so much and inspired me both to seek more deeply for answers and to question received wisdom; to my parents, for having imbued me with their love of the beauty and the power of the English language; and to all my family and friends, for their kind patience and understanding during the long gestation of this book.

Contents

Section IV: Staying Pain-Free, 199

Preface

As a neuromuscular therapist, my practice is focused on pain relief. Having had almost 30 years of chronic and sometimes disabling back pain before I found its cause and figured out how to rid myself of it permanently, I know only too well the havoc and torment that such unremitting pain can cause, and one of my greatest joys in life is helping others to get out of pain.

My job is first to analyze structure and function in my clients' bodies, note any distortions in structure (for example, a low left shoulder, a high pelvis on the right, a forward head posture), and then address the soft tissue components (muscles, tendons, and ligaments) that can be contributing to those distortions and creating the resultant pain. However, I feel that the second and perhaps more important part of my job is thoroughly to educate the people I treat regarding the structural causes of their pain conditions and how they themselves can help reduce or even totally eliminate such pain in the future. I think it is usually unnecessary, and therefore wrong, for people to be dependent on someone else for long-term relief from musculoskeletal pain, so I try to give each person who comes to me the tools that he or she needs to become and remain as self-sufficient as possible in controlling and preventing pain.

Time and again I have seen people greatly reduce their pain levels, and in many cases become pain-free, once they understood what was causing their pain and how to avoid or counteract it. In the course of explaining this information to each new client who came in, I realized that teaching this approach to people one at a time was incredibly inefficient and that, because there probably would never be enough trained therapists in the world to treat all of the millions of people in pain, I needed to think of how best to convey these simple and effective pain relief principles to a wider audience.

Of the several possibilities that came to mind, writing it all down in a compact, inexpensive, and widely available format seemed the best way to help the greatest number of people. So, with great trepidation, I sat down to undertake the Herculean task of clearly and concisely setting down in writing the volume of information I have so easily rattled off verbally for years to so many hundreds of clients and students.

As you read this book, please keep in mind three very important points:

1. This book is not intended to provide medical advice or to diagnose or treat any medical condition. The exercises, stretches, ideas, and recommendations presented are those that I have found helpful and effective in restoring proper muscular balance, creating good postural alignment, and reducing or eliminating pain. However, although they are time tested, based on common sense and sound principles, and have worked for many people, they may not be appropriate for you or your particular condition. Accordingly, it is recommended that you obtain the approval of your physician or other primary healthcare provider before beginning any exercise or stretching program. Also, there are other causes of pain, such as injury and disease, that are not within the scope of this book and may require other forms of treatment. These conditions should be ruled out by your physician or other primary healthcare provider before you begin this program.

2. Even the best book is of no use if its advice is not followed. I'm always amazed when a client comes back for his next appointment and says, "I don't think this is working. I still have the same amount of pain," only to find, upon questioning, that he hasn't done any of the things I suggested. It's pretty simple, really: If we don't follow the directions in the cookbook, it's hardly surprising if the recipe doesn't turn out as expected.

3. It takes some time to achieve results. Rome wasn't built in a day, and, although minor problems of recent onset many times do resolve quickly, most chronic musculoskeletal pain, except in cases where the pain has originated from traumatic injury or disease, is the result of long-standing postural distortion caused by our habitual postures and activities, whether or not we are conscious of them. Persistent or chronic pain caused by years or decades of poor posture can hardly be expected to resolve overnight, yet if you understand the simple principles outlined in this book and employ them properly and consistently, over time you will be able to greatly reduce or even eliminate many of your pain complaints, as well as to help prevent new ones.

So many people suffer with pain needlessly when some simple self-care could help restore them to happy, healthy, productive lives. In addition, along with their physical suffering, the ever-increasing burden of rising healthcare costs often adds to their misery. To me, there is no higher calling than helping a fellow human being to get out of pain, and I would consider it a genuine privilege to assist you in reducing or eliminating your chronic or persistent pain. All I ask in return is that you share in this work by spreading the word to others that *a lot of pain is optional*, and that there *is* a way out. Once you know, it is important for you to help others to know.

Total Commitment:
Dedicating Yourself to Pain Relief

Health can be no more obtained by payment of gold than a child can purchase his education: no sum of money can teach the pupil to write, he must learn of himself, guided by an experienced teacher. And so it is with health.

—Dr. Edward Bach

Tony was only 21 and still in college when surgeons shaved one of his lumbar disks to relieve the excruciating pain in his right leg. When he came to me shortly after the surgery had healed, I checked his psoas major muscles, deep in his abdomen, and found the left one rock-hard and tight. Knowing that Tony was a devoted "gym rat," I asked about his workout routine and especially whether he did hanging leg raises, supporting himself on his elbows while lifting his legs out in front of him. "Yeah, I really like those," he answered, to which I replied, "That's great, but if you keep doing them, in two or three years you'll probably need another disk shaved. Then, a few years after that, when a third disk acts up and you need another operation, they'll probably want to fuse your lumbar spine." Without a moment's hesitation, he said, "I will do *anything* to avoid ever having that kind of pain again."

Those were the magic words I was hoping to hear. That attitude of absolute dedication to pain relief meant that Tony had a great chance at avoiding future pain and surgery. I released the extreme tension in his psoas muscles, then changed his beloved workout routine to avoid retightening his psoas muscles and to keep his overall musculature balanced. In the eight years since, he's remained pain-free.

Pain is incredibly common in our society. A Gallup survey released on April 6, 2000, of 1,000 male and 1,002 female Americans aged 18 years and older stated that 89 percent reported having pain at least once a month and that 15 percent of those who had pain monthly said the pain was severe. Some studies have indicated that as much as 40 percent of the population lives with persistent or chronic pain, and the cost of that pain, in both financial and human terms, is staggering. Businesses lose billions of dollars each year as a result of employee absenteeism, increased healthcare premiums, and employee errors due to the distraction of chronic pain. Many sufferers' lives are radically changed, sometimes apparently forever; they frequently lose income due to time taken off from work and all too often lose jobs they can no longer perform; many lose spouses or friends who can no longer deal with the emotional toll that being with someone in severe, constant pain often takes; and perhaps the greatest loss is the human potential that is never expressed because of the crushing burden of unremitting pain.

There are, of course, many causes of pain, and this book does not deal with them all. However, it has been estimated that as much as 80 percent of all pain is musculoskeletal in origin, and it is that huge portion of pain that this book addresses. The soft tissues of our bodies—our muscles, tendons, and ligaments—are subject to a wide range of stresses and strains as a result of even the most innocent-seeming of our daily activities, and these stresses, if not detected and corrected, can build up until finally they result in perceived pain. If the stresses that produced the pain continue to remain uncorrected, that pain can become chronic or persistent, with effects ranging from the merely annoying to the disabling and even life-threatening.

It doesn't have to be this way. Serious injury or disease aside, the great bulk of the remainder of musculoskeletal pain is a result of our lack of awareness of those underlying stresses and how they occur in the course of our daily lives. If we once understand the physical consequences of our habitual actions and postures, we can use that newfound awareness to make changes in our daily routines and to counteract those pain-generating effects. In short, we can take ourselves out of pain.

One of the concepts I stress when I teach this work is finding the "root cause" of the pain. When we take pain relievers or muscle-relaxing medications to ease musculoskeletal pain, we only mask the symptoms without finding and addressing the root cause of the problem. Similarly, many of us know people who have had one or more surgeries to relieve pain and dysfunction but who have found themselves with just as much pain and dysfunction after the surgery. Although clearly many surgeries are both necessary and successful, there are obviously others that are not, and here again it is helpful to see if we can discover a hitherto undetected root cause. Even if a neuromuscular therapist finds a trigger point in a muscle that is causing referred pain, treats it successfully, and relieves the person's pain, the root cause still has not been found. It is important to know *why* that muscle became so stressed—that is, what caused it to create the trigger point in the first place. If that root cause has not been discovered and corrected, the pain will sooner or later recur and the problem will continue unless and until the root cause is finally resolved. In my experience, the root cause for the majority of chronic pain problems, other than those caused by disease or trauma, lies in our postural distortions, and it is with the nature of these distortions and how to correct them that this book deals.

For those who are so inclined, there are dozens, perhaps hundreds, of scientific books and papers dealing with the subject of pain in a highly technical and theoretical manner; this book is not one of them. Although a very limited amount of technical information will be necessary to understand the principles involved, I have tried to make this book as clear, simple, and understandable as possible. The explanations are the same ones I have used and refined in explaining these principles time after time to hundreds of clients and students from all walks of life, and those explanations have proven easy for people to grasp and use successfully. I think you'll find the study of the human body fascinating and, especially if you suffer from pain, potentially life-changing.

Ready? Then let's begin.

Philosophy 101

Set out here are a few basic principles that underlie the philosophy of this book. These principles should be read, understood, and constantly kept in mind, not only while reading this book, but every day of your life. If you do so, both your outlook and your health will almost certainly improve.

▶ **Your body doesn't come with an owner's manual, but that doesn't mean you can get away without regular maintenance any more than your car can.**

Just as with your car, if you neglect your body you'll wind up with major, and often very expensive, problems; keep your car and your body well maintained and they'll give you many years of excellent, trouble-free service.

▶ **When it comes to staying well, you are your own primary healthcare provider.**

It's not Dr. So-and-So or the XYZ Clinic; it's *you*. Think about it: No one on the face of this planet cares more about your health than you do. Too often in this society people go passively, hat in hand, to their various healthcare providers, never questioning things they don't understand and blindly following advice even on those occasions when they instinctively sense that that advice may not be correct. Naturally, it is wise to seek the counsel of various healthcare providers—physicians, chiropractors, dentists, neuromuscular therapists, physical therapists, and so on—and to follow that counsel when it seems sound and correct to you to do so. Their advice may be very caring and based on years of imposing training and experience, but ultimately these people all work for *you*. If you get the real help, good advice, and excellent service you're entitled to, great! By all means, keep those providers on your healthcare team, respect them, and continue to solicit their advice. However, if you don't get the first-class help, advice, and service you need (and are paying for), fire the unsatisfactory providers, then seek out and hire new ones who will give you the assistance, answers, and respect you deserve. Remember, though, that *you* are ultimately in charge, and when you really take charge of your own healthcare instead of passively handing over the control to others, you'll be amazed at how energizing and empowering it can be. Interestingly enough, I think you'll also discover that your health will improve as well.

▶ **You, and you alone, live in your body, and you alone are responsible for its daily care and upkeep.**

You see your doctor or other healthcare providers only occasionally, and only for a brief visit; the rest of the time you're on your own. Only *you* can decide what and how much you eat and drink, whether and how much you exercise, and whether and how much you work, play, and sleep. This responsibility is yours, and yours alone, and if you neglect these things you have no one to blame but yourself if your body therefore gets sick or becomes painful. In short: **There is no substitute for personal responsibility if you want to stay healthy and avoid pain.**

▶ **Poor posture produces pain.**

Whatever we do habitually/constantly/repeatedly determines which muscles we chronically tighten or lengthen, and therefore our postural distortions and the resultant pain. As you'll soon learn, even apparently harmless activities like sitting, if done to excess, can cause postural distortion and pain.

▸ **Because we necessarily use or neglect certain muscles to the exclusion of others in the course of our work or other daily activities, we have no choice but to counterbalance the muscular effects of our daily activities if we want to avoid postural distortion and pain.**

Obviously we can't just give up our jobs or put the rest of our lives on hold. We can, however, counterbalance the effects of those daily activities with a properly tailored stretching and exercise program designed to correct our postural distortions, thereby minimizing or eliminating pain. This book will show you how to create that program for yourself.

▸ **Balanced exercise programs only work for posturally balanced bodies.**

Although a balanced exercise program can have many valuable health benefits, equally strengthening unbalanced muscle groups only further locks the body into its dysfunctional posture. In fact, strengthening the wrong muscles, however unintentionally, can sometimes cause the very pain we're trying to avoid. Virtually all of us have unbalanced bodies, so we need workout programs specifically tailored for each of us to properly counterbalance the unique muscular effects brought about by our individual lives and occupations. Your exercise and stretching program needs to be as unique as you are.

▸ **If you believe that you will always have pain, you almost certainly will.**

It will become a self-fulfilling prophecy. Ask yourself honestly if you can envision yourself without pain. Remember: We cannot create what we cannot envision.

▸ **You have the ability to reduce or eliminate your musculoskeletal pain and change your life.**

Whether you use this ability is up to you. The purpose of this book is to put into your hands the techniques to control or eliminate your current pain and to keep from incurring avoidable pain in the future. This book will give you the basic tools; all you need after that is your own effort and determination.

▸ **Masking your pain with medication is not the same as resolving your pain problem.**

Pain-relieving medications can be a great help when someone is suffering from intense pain, and when used appropriately they are truly a blessing. However, they are not designed to correct the original cause of the pain, but rather to keep us from feeling the effects of that cause. Because pain is our body's way of telling us that something is wrong, using pain relievers to turn down the volume doesn't change the fact that we need to listen to the body's message and take appropriate action before even greater pain and dysfunction result.

▶ **Getting yourself out of pain is naturally rewarding, but it is a process that takes work, commitment, and unflinching determination.**

The story is told of a young man who asked a great philosopher to teach him wisdom. Quickly sizing up the young man, the philosopher instructed him to kneel by the edge of a nearby stream and look deeply into the water. As soon as the young man knelt and leaned over to look into the stream, the philosopher pushed the young man's head under water and held it there. The young man struggled hard to escape, but the philosopher was both strong and relentless. Finally the philosopher released his hold on the young man, who came up gasping for air. The philosopher then quietly told him, "When you crave wisdom as much as you craved that breath of air, you will be ready to learn." If you crave true healing and pain relief as much as that young man craved that next breath, your commitment and determination can carry you farther than you ever thought possible.

Section I

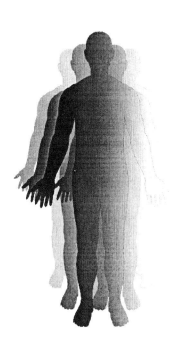

Understanding Your Pain

Chapter 1

Pain Basics:
Learning the Laws of the Body

A dynamic businessman, Mark suffered from terrible headaches and tight shoulder muscles on his left side, but when I learned that he often drove 10 hours a day with his right elbow on the center console of his car and his left hand on the top of the steering wheel, I instantly knew why he hurt so badly. I explained to Mark that the body has laws by which it operates and which he had unwittingly violated. I helped him understand that the Righting Reflex instinctively corrects our posture to keep the head upright and the eyes level, so that when he continuously leaned to the right during his long drives, the muscles of his left shoulder were in constant contraction to hold his head upright. Not only that, but when muscles are in a shortened position for any length of time, they tend to adapt by remaining shorter, thus causing his left shoulder to remain higher even when he wasn't driving, as well as stimulating muscular trigger points that referred pain up his neck and directly into his familiar headache area. Once I released his contracted muscles and he corrected his driving posture, Mark was able to remain pain-free.

The laws that govern the body are natural laws, and unlike manmade laws, where violation of the law brings varying results, natural laws always bring about the same result every time the laws are violated in the same way. If someone violates a manmade law against theft, say by stealing a loaf of bread, the result may vary from a warning or probation to jail time, or in some countries surgical removal of a hand, or even death. When someone violates natural law, however, the effect never varies; no matter how many times people step off the top of 50-story skyscrapers, the effect of gravity is always the same, regardless of the country in which the skyscraper is located. They may argue with the law of gravity all the way to the ground, they may call it unfair or inconvenient, but the law continues to work exactly the same way each time, regardless of their opinion of it.

Consequently, if we want to learn how to take charge of the pain in our bodies, we need to know the natural laws that govern its operation. Annie Besant, a noted writer of the late 19th and early 20th century, once put it beautifully: "Nature is conquered by obedience." Although it may at first seem contradictory to think of conquering something by obeying it, a little thought will demonstrate the truth and wisdom of that statement.

Let's say we're driving a car around a sharp curve. The laws of physics tell us that centrifugal force will tend to make the car travel in a straight line and go off the road, rather than following the curve we are attempting to steer through. However, the laws of physics also tell us that several factors will determine whether we stay on the road as we go around the curve, including the friction of our tires against the road, the degree to which the road is banked, the speed of our car (which determines the amount of centrifugal force created), the condition of the road surface, the condition of our tires, and so on. If we attempt to negotiate the curve in a driving rainstorm, which reduces the traction of our tires, we must take the laws of nature into account by slowing down on the slick surface to reduce the centrifugal force generated by our car, or else we will slide off the road and crash.

Similarly, when man first attempted powered flight, all kinds of flying contraptions were designed, and all met with dismal failure, because they were not designed in accordance with the natural laws governing wing shape, lift, and the like. Once those laws were obeyed and proper wing shapes created, man was able to conquer the air and fly freely at will.

It's clearly important, then, to know the natural laws that govern the body so that we can work in obedience to them in getting and keeping ourselves free from pain. If we ignore those laws, then all our efforts to get out of pain will ultimately crash and burn, just as cars or planes do that are not designed and operated in accordance with the natural laws that govern them. Following are some key laws of the body we need to know.

Muscles

The basic law that underlies muscle function is simple: Muscles only contract. Muscles can't push anything; they can only pull. What makes effective movement possible is that muscles work in opposing pairs or groups on opposite sides of every joint. For example, when you want to flex or bend your elbow, you use (among others) the biceps muscle in the front of the upper arm, an elbow flexor, meaning that it flexes or bends the elbow joint. When you want to extend or straighten your elbow joint, you use the triceps muscle in the back of your upper arm, the opposing extensor. Knowing how muscles work enables you to figure out which muscles may be causing a particular pain problem by seeing which ones are in a tight or contracted state.

Adaptive Shortening and Stretch Weakening

This concept explains how muscles adapt to the demands placed upon them. Simply put, if a muscle is kept in a shortened state, with the muscle ends brought closer together, the muscle adapts to that shortened state and tends to remain shortened, as well as increasing in tonus or resistance to stretch. The opposite is also true: If a muscle is kept in a lengthened state, with the muscle ends farther apart than normal, the tonus is decreased (the muscle becomes less resistant to stretch) and the muscle tends to remain lengthened or stretched. Because muscles work in opposing groups, if the muscles on one side of a joint are shortened and stronger while the muscles on the other side of the joint are stretched and weaker, clearly the stronger muscles are going to win out and distort the alignment of the body at that joint. As we'll soon discover, adaptive shortening is a vital key in understanding how pain conditions can develop not only when we're engaging in apparently harmless activity, but even during periods of inactivity.

Gravity

Yes, our old friend gravity is important in understanding how pain is caused in our bodies. Gravity is the force exerted upon all things by the earth's mass, and it tends to pull all things toward the center of the earth. This force is acting upon our bodies at all times, and when we have good posture the force of gravity is carried correctly through our bones into the earth. When our posture is poor, however, our muscles have to stay in constant contraction in order to counteract the force of gravity and try to keep us upright, as a result of which gravity can put a terrible strain on our muscles, causing a great deal of pain and dysfunction. (We'll cover this in greater detail in Chapter 2.)

Center of Gravity

In addition to understanding in general the effects of gravity in forcing our muscles to compensate for our poor posture, it's helpful to grasp the concept of the center of gravity. Any object that has mass has what is called a center of gravity, meaning that point that is the precise center of the object's mass.

"The center of gravity is defined as the single point of a body about which every particle of its mass is equally distributed.... If the body were suspended (or supported) at this point, the body would be perfectly balanced. Each body behaves as if its entire mass were acting or being acted upon at its center of gravity."[1]

To illustrate this, let's assume we have a vertical post or support, infinitely strong so that it can support whatever weight we put on it, and that the top of the post tapers to a tiny pinpoint. Now let's assume we take a board that is 3 feet long by 1 foot wide and of a uniform one inch thickness and mass throughout. If we measure the midline between the two ends and between the two sides, where those two lines cross is the exact center of gravity of the board, and, if we position the board so that this center of gravity is exactly on the point of our post, it will be perfectly balanced. If the center of gravity of the board is even the slightest bit off to any side of the supporting pinpoint, the effect of gravity will cause the board to topple to that side.

If you want to try this at home, take a dinner plate (preferably unbreakable!) and try to balance it on the tip of your index finger. When you find the point where the plate balances perfectly on the tip of your finger, you've found the plate's center of gravity. If you now shift the plate even a tiny fraction of an inch in any direction, it will fall toward that side.

The exact same principle applies to anything that has mass, whether it's a coffee cup, a zebra, a diesel locomotive, or a human being. Unfortunately, it's a little more difficult to determine the center of gravity for irregularly shaped objects such as these, but it can be done. For a typical human being standing upright, the center of gravity is located in the midline of the body just anterior to (in front of) the second sacral vertebra; put more simply, it's usually about 3 inches or so below the navel and roughly in the center of the pelvis.

How does our center of gravity relate to our pain? When our muscles or skeletal system are out of balance and tend to allow our pelvis (and therefore our center of gravity) to move too far forward, backward, or to one side, other muscles are forced to compensate by contracting constantly to prevent us from toppling forward, backward, or sideways. As mentioned above, muscles that have to contract constantly are a prolific source of pain in our bodies.

Righting Reflex

The Righting Reflex is actually a group of related reflexes that enables you to maintain your body in an upright position, an obvious advantage if you want to remain functional. Using receptors in the balance center of the inner ear, the eyes, and other areas of the body, the Righting Reflex instinctively corrects your body's position in order to keep your head upright and your eyes level with the horizon, as well as keep your body's center of gravity safely within the base of support provided by your feet. Having a good grasp of the Righting Reflex will enable us to understand why certain muscles instinctively tighten, thereby causing pain, as well as why certain postural abnormalities naturally cause scoliosis, a lateral or sideways curvature of the spine, to occur.

Does all this talk of laws sound a bit complex or intimidating at the moment? If so, don't worry; you don't need to memorize them all, and there's not going to be a surprise quiz. Although they are vital to understanding how poor posture creates pain in the body, you'll soon become quite comfortable with these laws as we progress, and before long you'll find yourself referring to them as if you were an old hand at it.

All set, then? Okay, let's find out what posture's all about.

Chapter 2

Posture Basics:
Recognizing the Good, the Bad,
and the Ugly

When Roger, a construction worker with chest and arm muscles made strong through years of hard physical work, first came in, he had been experiencing chest and arm pain, along with difficulty in taking a really deep breath, yet the doctors had tested and retested his heart and lungs, only to pronounce them perfectly healthy. A glance at his shoulders, however, explained the source of his distress. His chest muscles had become so strong and overdeveloped that his shoulders had been pulled forward, allowing his chest muscles to shorten and tighten further, thus restricting his deep breathing and activating trigger points in his chest muscles that fired into his chest, shoulder, and arms. With a properly designed therapy program, Roger was able to stretch his chest muscles and strengthen his back muscles, thus restoring his shoulders to their normal position and relieving his pain.

What is good posture? Although many of us have some general ideas of what constitutes good posture (for example, sit up straight, don't slouch, and so on), very few people know that posture is actually something that can be scientifically evaluated. The vertical lines on the postural chart shown in Figure 2-1 are based on the research of Dr. Peter Bachin and are designed to show the correct alignment of the body in a standing position. If you look at the vertical line that runs through the center of the front, back, and side views, you'll see that in each case it divides the body perfectly in half, both side to side and front to back. That vertical line is the line of gravity, and the illustrations represent the alignment our bodies should have with gravity when we are standing with perfect posture.

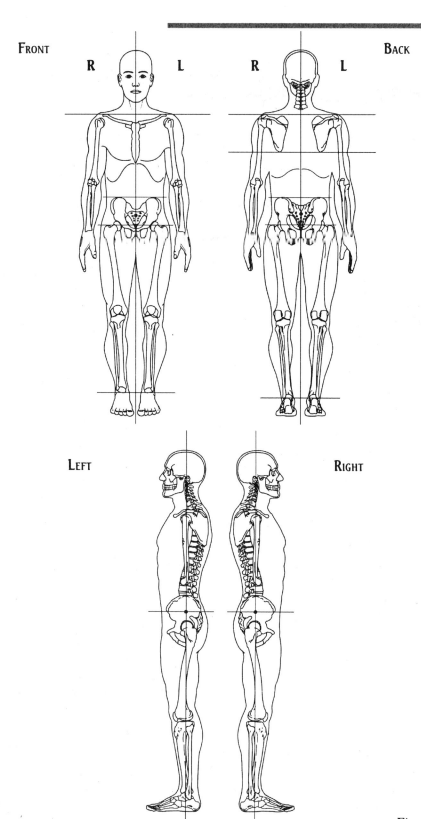

FRONT   R   L   R   L   BACK

LEFT   RIGHT

Figure 2-1

A few terms need to be introduced here. If you look at the front and back views and imagine an ultra-thin metal sheet, like a huge blade, dividing the body exactly down the middle (along the vertical lines) into equal right and left halves, that sheet is said to be on what is called the midsagittal plane. Likewise, if you look at the side view and imagine a similar sheet running straight through the body from the near side to the far side and dividing the body into front and back halves along the vertical line, that sheet would be on what is called the coronal plane. Finally, if you turn that imaginary sheet so that it is horizontal and pass it through the body horizontally at any point—at the level of the ankles, hips, shoulders, or ears—that sheet is said to be on a horizontal plane. It's important to note that, although there can be an infinite number of horizontal planes through the body, the midsagittal plane and coronal plane are unique and occur only along the vertical lines shown.

So what does all that mean? Simply this: When we are perfectly aligned on the midsagittal plane (not tilting either left or right) and on the coronal plane (not tilted forward or backward), and if we are level at all matching points on both sides of the body (knees, hips, shoulders, etc.), then we have perfect posture. When the body has perfect posture, it is precisely balanced right and left, forward and backward, and the weight of the body is properly carried by the bones into the earth. The job of bones is to carry weight, whereas the job of muscles is to move bones; consequently, because the bones are doing their job, the majority of the muscles (all but the few muscles needed to keep the body stable) are free to relax until needed for movement.

This is an important point. Healthy muscle tissue at rest is not tight and contracted, but firm, supple, and relaxed, and should remain so until called on for action, at which time the muscles contract to produce the desired movement. Once the movement is over, the muscles relax and the bones return to their original neutral position. However, muscles are not designed for constant, prolonged contraction, and this is what happens in postural distortion.

Let's take the simple example of lifting a 5-pound weight (if you're unusually small or large, adjust the amount of the weight accordingly). As you hold the weight at your side and flex your arm at the elbow to bring the weight up in front of you so that you're holding it with your palm up, you have just used your elbow flexor muscles. Assuming you're of average build and strength, and that the weight is properly sized for you, you should be able to lift the weight this way and hold it there for a brief time without tiring your elbow flexor muscles unduly. Now imagine having to hold it in that position for, say, eight hours continuously. Instantly, you know intuitively what will happen: Your arm muscles, no matter how strong, would soon tire and begin to ache, ultimately becoming painful and, finally, going into spasm. In fact, even if you flex your elbow with your hand holding nothing but air, just the weight of your forearm and hand will start to create the ache/pain/spasm response if you hold them up that way for too long. This ache/pain/spasm response due to muscle overload is incredibly common and you'll see in the next chapter how this kind of constant contraction can be the source of a lot of your chronic pain.

What is postural distortion? In order to answer that properly, we need first to make a distinction between postural distortion and poor posture. We have poor posture any time we sit or stand so that the body is not exactly aligned on the midsagittal, coronal, and horizontal planes just described. If this poor posture is or becomes our "normal" posture—not our ideal posture, mind you, but the posture our body naturally assumes when at rest in the sitting or standing position—we now have postural distortion. Mary may sit or stand with poor posture occasionally, but if when she straightens up and sits or stands in her normal posture she is aligned properly on all three planes, she does not have postural distortion. However, if Mary straightens up into her normal posture and she still slumps forward a bit and her right shoulder is low, she has postural distortion. In effect, poor posture may be only occasional or momentary, but postural distortion is chronic and is often caused by persistent poor posture.

For example, if your pelvis always tilts to the left or right while standing, the result is postural distortion because your pelvis has tilted off the horizontal plane and your upper body has moved off the midsagittal plane to one side. Let's say your pelvis tilts to the left, which can be caused by many factors, including a fallen arch in the left foot or an anatomically short left leg. The result of this is that your weight is shifted more onto your left leg, and your head and shoulders would normally tend to lean to the left as well. This causes a problem, for if we slump or tilt in any way, our bodies are no longer balanced and able to properly carry our weight through our bones, so our muscles have to compensate by contracting to try to keep the body upright. In the simple example we're using here, if your pelvis tilts to the left, thereby tilting the upper body and head to the left, the muscles on the right side of your body and neck naturally tighten up in order to keep you as erect as possible.

The same thing happens if your pelvis tilts too far anterior (forward), a very widespread problem in our society. Among the most common causes of this distortion are repeated sitting for long periods of time, obesity, pregnancy, and wearing high-heeled shoes or cowboy boots. (We'll talk more about each of these causes later.) Because an anteriorly tilted pelvis forces the upper body to lean forward, your low back muscles have no choice but to compensate by pulling your spine upright, or else you'd always walk around leaning over, bent forward at the hips.

Why does your body automatically compensate for postural distortion? The answer lies in two of those laws we talked about in Chapter 1. First of all, the Righting Reflex instinctively tries to correct your posture to ensure that you stay upright with your eyes level with the horizon. If your pelvis tilts to one side, your spine and head will naturally tilt to that side, too, causing your eyes to tilt with respect to the horizon. Because remaining for long in this position will adversely affect your balance, the Righting Reflex instinctively tightens the muscles on your opposite side in order to try to make your eyes level and bring your spine and head back toward the midsagittal plane as much as possible.

The other law that's involved in this process is gravity, and particularly the idea of the center of gravity. Remember the statement from Chapter 1: "Each body behaves as if its entire mass were acting or being acted upon at its center of gravity." That tells us that as long as the center of gravity of a body is located within the area of its support (in this case, between your feet), it will be stable and won't fall. Look at Figure 2-2. The center of gravity (shown by the black dot) is in the back of the lower abdomen, just in front of the upper sacrum. As long as this point stays between your feet, you won't fall to either side, which is why a wide stance is so stable. However, if you place your feet in a straight line, one exactly behind the other (as if walking a tightrope), you'll quickly find that, because you've narrowed your base of support, this position is very unstable and that, if you let your center of gravity move even the least bit outside your supporting feet to either side, you'll fall to that side.

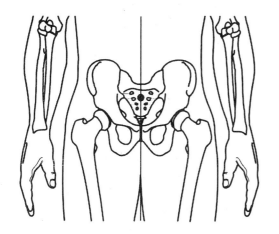
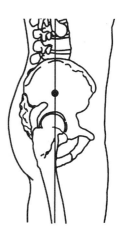

Figure 2-2

The same is true with tilting forward and backward. In ideal posture, the center of gravity should be located above a point just slightly in front of the ankle bone, as shown by the vertical line in the side view in Figure 2-1. However, if your pelvis tilts too far forward, which is naturally accompanied by a forward tilt of the legs from the ankle, this moves your center of gravity forward so that instead of being approximately over your ankle it is closer to being over the balls of your feet. Similarly, if your pelvis tilts posteriorly (backward), your center of gravity moves back toward your heels.

The absolute best way to understand the effects of postural distortion is to duplicate the distortion in our own bodies or, if it's a distortion we already have, to increase its severity. This also has the side benefit of helping us to develop a lot of sympathy and compassion for those greatly affected by postural distortion.

To experience the muscular effects of a tilted pelvis, stand with your feet about shoulder-width apart and your hands grasping your hips, fingers in front, thumbs in back. Using your hands to help if necessary, tilt your pelvis forward (your fingers will be pressing down in front, your thumbs pressing up in back) and hold that position. Wait for a few moments and you'll notice that your entire body seems gradually to drift forward into that same tilt, and that your weight is now more on the balls of your feet as your center of gravity moves forward. You'll also notice that you instinctively start to tighten certain muscles along the back side of your body in order to pull yourself back, because, if your body drifts forward enough to allow your center of gravity to move past the balls of your feet, you'll fall on your face. This instinctive tightening of your posterior muscles is exactly what your body does if you have an anteriorly rotated pelvis.

Now try tilting your pelvis posteriorly by turning your hips back the other way (fingers pressing up in front, thumbs pressing down in back). Hold this for a few moments and you'll feel your weight drifting back over your heels as your center of gravity moves backward. Here, too, your body has to tighten certain muscles in the front of your body in order to keep you from falling on your back.

To feel what a lateral or sideways pelvic tilt feels like, put a book or stack of magazines about ½-inch thick on the floor, then stand with your left foot on the book and your right foot on the floor next to the book so that the insides of your feet are touching, or very nearly so. As you assume this position and let your weight settle, you should feel your pelvis tilt to the right and your upper body compensate by tilting back to the left. (If by chance you actually feel more stable with the left foot on the book, there's a good chance that you may have a shorter left leg, but we'll deal with that subject a little later on.)

In sum, as long as your center of gravity is located above a point that is between your feet, and between your heels and the balls of your feet, you'll be stable. If it moves outside that base of support by even a fraction of an inch, you'll fall over. As a result, your body instinctively tightens muscles to pull you back from the edges of this base of support to keep your center of gravity as close as possible to its ideal position.

Okay, so your muscles tighten and keep you from toppling over. What does that have to do with your chronic muscular pain? Simply put, everything. Remember the example we used earlier of lifting the 5-pound weight? Lifting the weight briefly was no problem for healthy muscles, but having to hold it there for a prolonged time caused the muscles to become tired, then painful, and perhaps even to go into spasm. This is because muscles are not intended to contract continuously; they are designed to contract long enough to move bones into some new position, hold them there briefly if necessary, and then relax until needed again. Keep in mind that the job of bones is to support weight, whereas the job of muscles is to move bones; consequently, when muscles are forced to do the job of bone (that is, support weight) for a long time, they become like bone: stiff, hard, and tight. This can lead not only to local pain and spasm in the muscle itself, but also to referred pain in other parts of the body.

Sudden muscle spasm is in many cases a result of this habitual overloading of those muscles due to poor posture. Think about how many times you've heard people say something along the lines of, "I sneezed in the shower and my back went into spasm" or "I reached for the salt at the dinner table and my back locked up." I think we can safely agree that sneezing and reaching for the salt shaker are not inherently back-destroying activities, so it's clear that these actions simply were the trigger mechanisms that set off existing muscular problems. When muscles are in constant contraction in order to compensate for postural distortion, that constant tension can build up until the muscles are just on the verge of going into spasm, so that all it takes is some apparently inconsequential action to send the muscles into spasm, just as a falling pebble can start an avalanche if the conditions are right.

Referred pain is caused by what are known as "trigger points" in the dysfunctional muscles. A trigger point is an area of hyperirritability in a muscle or other soft tissues that is not only locally tender when compressed or otherwise stressed, but can also refer pain or other symptoms to other parts of the body. Although pain is perhaps the most common of the referred symptoms, an active trigger point can also cause such other referred sensations as numbness, tingling, sensations of heat or cold, or goose flesh. Frequently these symptoms are referred to areas of the body quite some distance away from the site of the trigger point and often mimic pains produced by other causes, sometimes resulting in incorrect diagnoses.

For example, there are muscles on the sides of the pelvis and in the low back whose trigger point referrals mimic the aching leg pain of sciatica, and trigger points in muscles underneath the shoulder blade and in the forearm can sometimes refer into the wrist, causing pain that is occasionally mistaken for the onset of carpal tunnel syndrome. Several muscles in the neck and shoulder area refer into the head and eyes to create chronic headache pain, and the referrals from a number of neck and mouth muscles can cause ringing in the ears, vertigo, dizziness, or balance problems. Additionally, there are muscles in the face, head, neck, and shoulder that can refer into the jaw, the TMJ (the temporomandibular joint or jaw joint), and even into specific teeth.

Barbara was a classic example of this last condition. When she first came to my office, she had had chronic pain in her right jaw and teeth for more than 20 years, along with frequent devastating headaches. She had lost track of how many thousands of dollars she had spent on extensive dental treatments over the years in a desperate search for relief, but all to no avail. No sooner did I start working the upper trapezius muscle at the top of her right shoulder than she exclaimed, "That's making my jaw pain come back!" Bingo. That was a sure sign that we'd found, if not the only source of her pain, at least one of the primary sources. The same thing happened when I worked a muscle in the side of her neck; there was an instant referral of pain into her jaw, recreating her all too familiar pain pattern. In addition, both muscles also re-created her headache pain as well. By the time we finished the session, her jaw no longer hurt and her headaches were almost gone.

Perhaps my "favorite" referrals, though, are those that mimic sciatica and arthritis. I'd like to have a five-dollar bill for every time a client has told me that he or she had sciatica on one side or arthritis in a certain joint, only to find after I worked the muscles that referred deep aching pain into the affected area that the "sciatica" or "arthritis" had magically disappeared. Although, of course, there are all too much genuine sciatica and arthritis, both painful and potentially crippling conditions, it is surprising how often clients with apparent sciatica or localized arthritis can be helped by relieving the trigger points that refer into those painful areas.

Such trigger points are frequently caused by muscular imbalances as the muscles react to postural distortion in accordance with the laws of the body discussed in Chapter 1, and I can tell you from years of both professional and personal experience that these referrals from trigger points in overstressed muscles constitute one of the major sources of chronic musculoskeletal pain. As a result, if you can eliminate or counteract the postural stress on your muscles, you can greatly reduce, or even eliminate, your chronic pain, and that's what this book is designed to teach you.

Now that you have a general idea of what postural distortion is, let's look at some important areas of the body and see how postural distortion in those areas can cause your pain.

Chapter 3

Pelvis Basics 1:
Rotating Forward and Backward

A hardworking nurse in a busy hospital, Liz spent much of her day either bent over patients in beds or sitting at a desk doing lots of paperwork. In both situations, she was in a hip-flexed posture for extended periods of time, so when in the course of doing her postural evaluation I found her pelvis rotated forward at an angle of 15 degrees, rather than in the normal range for females of 5 to 10 degrees, I was hardly surprised. Because this kind of rotation causes the muscles in the back, shoulder, and neck to tighten in order to try to hold the body erect, it was only natural that Liz had been suffering with lower and upper back pain, neck pain, and headaches for several years. After finishing the postural evaluation, I did some therapy on the tight hip flexor muscles that were holding her pelvis forward, then had her get off the treatment table and stand.

Her eyes widened in surprise as her body swayed backward and forward for a few moments, trying to adjust to its new, more upright posture. "Wow, this is amazing!" she exclaimed. "I can't tell you how much better I feel." Then, about 10 minutes after she left my office, the phone rang. It was Liz again, absolutely ecstatic, calling from her car to tell me, "I can't believe it. I actually walked from your office to my car with my weight back toward my heels, instead of on my toes, and even the car seat feels different now that my pelvis is back where it belongs. Thank you so much!"

Of all the areas of the body in which postural distortion can occur, by far the most important is the pelvis. If you look back at Figure 2-1, you'll see why this is so. The pelvis essentially consists of the sacrum in the middle, wedged tightly between the right and left halves of the pelvis. What's critical to note here is that when a person is standing the spine rests on the top surface of the sacrum, sometimes called the sacral base. (The sacrum is actually part of the spine, but for our present discussion it is clearer and more convenient to consider the sacrum as part of the pelvis.) This means that if the sacral base is tilted left or right, or forward or backward, or if it is rotated to the left or right, the spine will not rise properly from the sacrum and will have to be pulled back toward ideal alignment by constant muscular contraction, a rich source of muscular pain.

The correct alignment of the pelvis is so important because not only do all the muscles that attach to the pelvis have to adjust and compensate for any pelvic distortion, but the spine, which sits on the pelvis, bears much of the weight of the upper body and anything it carries. If you pick up something, whether it is a 100-pound barbell, a 40-pound child, or a 10-pound bag of groceries, the weight you are carrying is transmitted through your arms, shoulders, and upper torso to your spine, which in turn transmits that lifted weight, plus the weight of much of your upper body, to the sacrum. The sacrum, which sits between the two halves of the pelvis like a keystone in an arch, then transmits that weight through the two halves of the pelvis to the legs and into the ground.

Not only is the pelvis important because of its key role in supporting the upper body and transmitting weight to the legs, but it is also the center of movement in the body. All locomotion goes through the pelvis, and if the muscles that attach to your pelvis all stiffen up you can't run, walk, or even crawl. This is often seen in people who have been immobile for a long time, perhaps in a wheelchair during a long recovery from an injury or illness. The muscles around the pelvis have adapted to the hip-flexed position that the wheelchair imposes, so standing upright and walking freely can be very difficult at first until proper physical therapy is provided.

There are three possible movement distortions at the pelvis, as shown in Figure 3-1. The pelvis can tilt left or right, as shown in Figure 3-1a; it can rotate anteriorly or posteriorly, as shown in Figure 3-1b; and it can rotate laterally to the right or left, as shown in Figure 3-1c. Sure, you may say, this is all fine and nice to know, but how likely is it that any of this applies to me? Surprising as it may seem, extremely likely.

Contrary to our natural assumption that we are symmetrical beings, with our left and right sides exact mirror images of each other, the truth is that almost none of us are symmetrical. I have done postural evaluations on hundreds and hundreds of people and have yet to find anyone with perfect, or

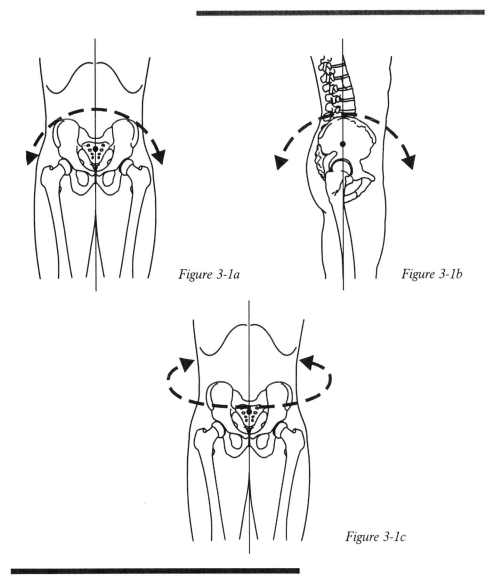

Figure 3-1a

Figure 3-1b

Figure 3-1c

even near-perfect, posture. Whether it's something congenital, such as a bone length discrepancy, or the result of an injury, or the accumulated effects of our habitual postures and activities, the simple truth is that virtually all of us have some postural distortion. In fact, when it comes to the three primary distortions of the pelvis, the vast majority of the people I've measured have all three distortions to some extent; occasionally I come across someone with only two of the three; and I can't remember anyone with only one of the three. Needless to say, the person with zero pelvic distortions—the foundation for perfect posture—has yet to darken my office door.

Let's look at the causes and effects of each of those three pelvic distortions. Perhaps the simplest and easiest to understand is forward and backward rotation. It is possible to measure this rotation, also known as the angle of pelvic inclination (API), by finding two landmarks, one each on the front and back of the pelvis, known as the anterior superior iliac spine (ASIS) and the posterior superior iliac spine (PSIS), drawing an imaginary line between them, and noting the angle that line of inclination forms with the horizontal. In a male pelvis, the normal range is from 0 degrees (exactly level) to 5 degrees anterior rotation; in a female pelvis the normal range is from 5 degrees to 10 degrees anterior, the difference being due to different hip structures in the two sexes. (See Figure 3-2.)

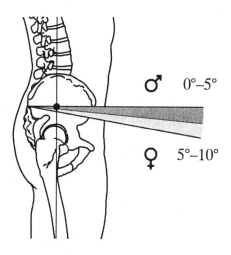

Figure 3-2

Posterior or backward rotation of the pelvis is not very common, although it certainly does happen. In a male, that means an API of less than 0 degrees (for example, -4 degrees, an actual backward tilt). In a female anything less than 5 degrees anterior (for example, 2 degrees) is considered to be posterior pelvic rotation. To experience this, stand erect with your feet parallel at about shoulder width, then tighten your hamstrings and gluteal (buttock) muscles to pull your pelvis down in back, bringing your tailbone down and forward. If you pay close attention, you'll notice that as your pelvis rotates backward, your lumbar curve (normally slightly concave when viewed from the back) flattens out, your knees buckle forward slightly, and your head and neck automatically come forward. The body does these things instinctively in order to help keep your center of gravity from moving too far posterior, to the point where you'd fall backward. This change tilts your neck so that you would actually face slightly downward if your body didn't instinctively correct for it, and, as you'll see shortly, this can be a major source of headaches and eye pain. Fortunately, as mentioned, posterior rotation is relatively uncommon.

However, it is extremely common to find the pelvis anteriorly rotated, so that the pelvis is tipped forward and the person is standing in a hip-flexed position. If you want to see what this feels like, keep your back straight, as if it were rigidly attached to your pelvis, and tip the pelvis forward by bending over slightly from the hips. You'll notice that this tilts your spine and your entire body forward, with the result that your body wants to fall forward. If you try it again slowly and pay very close attention, however, you'll notice that your low back muscles instinctively tighten to try to keep your spine upright and prevent you from falling on your face. If this tightening is only momentary, your muscles can take it in stride, but when these muscles have to stay in constant contraction every instant you are standing or walking—often for hours at a time—is it any wonder that you find yourself with an aching or painful low back?

Whether your posture is distorted or normal, if you want to really feel the effects of any distortion for yourself, you have to slightly exaggerate the distortion, then feel what it's like for the body to correct for it. As an example, let's say you're a woman with a 15-degree anterior pelvic rotation or a man with 10-degree anterior rotation, in each case 5 degrees greater than the normal range. Your awareness of your posture has gradually adapted over time so that your brain now accepts this posture as "correct," and only when you momentarily increase the distortion will your brain feel that something is now "wrong."

So to exaggerate the effects of anterior rotation, let's go back to the demonstration we used in Chapter 2, where you stand with your hands on your hips, fingers in front, thumbs in back, and, using your hands to help if necessary, tilt your pelvis forward (your fingers are pressing down in front, your thumbs pressing up in back). This naturally tilts your upper body forward and, because the body cannot function properly in this position, it instinctively tries to pull the spine back and stand erect. Now, being sure to hold your anteriorly tilted pelvis firmly in its new tilted position with your hands so it can't rotate back to its "normal" position, try to stand erect. You'll feel your low back muscles tighten up, and the greater the anterior rotation of the pelvis, the tighter the contraction in your back muscles when you try to stand upright.

In my experience, this anterior pelvic rotation is one of the most common causes of low back pain, and, if this is true of your pelvis, even the best back pills and pain relievers in the world will never permanently resolve your low back pain if that anterior rotation is not corrected. Not only does this anterior rotation cause low back pain, but the muscles that tighten and hold you in this position also tend to pull the vertebrae in your lumbar (low back) region together, thus squeezing the intervertebral disks between them. When the disks are squeezed by the pressure of the muscles on the vertebrae, it's only natural that they will start to bulge, in some cases even to the point where they rupture, and in severe cases these bulging or ruptured disks can put pressure on the nerve roots that come out of the spine or on the spinal cord itself, thereby causing pain down one or both legs. Although disk surgery may then remove the immediate cause of the leg pain, what's going to prevent the next disk above or below the injured disk from eventually suffering the same fate? Clearly, we need to release the tight muscles and correct the postural distortion in order to resolve the root cause of the problem or the pain and dysfunction will just continue.

As mentioned in the last chapter, there are several causes of anterior pelvic rotation, but perhaps the most common is repeated sitting for long periods of time. Scientists tell us that it took human beings more than 20 million years to adapt successfully to walking upright; we are now designed and built to be upright, active beings. The trouble is, though, that ever since the Industrial Revolution we've been trying to figure out every way possible to sit down! We glory now in our ability to sit at our desks and perform all kinds of functions with our computers, telephones, and faxes without ever having to get up from our chairs, yet that very immobility is causing a veritable epidemic of back pain, neck pain, and headaches.

Remember our discussion in Chapter 1 of the Law of Adaptive Shortening? Essentially, it says that if a muscle is kept in a shortened state, with the muscle ends brought closer together, the muscle adapts to that shortened state and tends to remain shortened, as well as increasing in tonus or resistance to stretch, and this process helps to explain a lot of chronic pain complaints. To illustrate this, let's say that you're an office worker and that you sit at your desk eight hours a day in the course of your job. (Keep in mind, though, that the same applies to anyone who maintains a hip-flexed position for long periods of time, including long-haul truck drivers, equestrians, motorcycle riders, TV watchers, speed skaters, and so on.)

As you go to sit down in your desk chair to begin your day, you have to bend at the hips in order to fit into the right angle formed by the back and seat of the chair. As your hips flex to approximately a 90-degree angle, the ends of your hip flexor muscles are brought closer together. (The hip flexor muscles are the ones that enable you to lift your knee toward your chest or, alternatively, to perform a true sit-up in which your lumbar spine and sacrum come off the floor and move toward your thigh bones.) As described by the

Law of Adaptive Shortening, because the ends of the hip flexor muscles just got closer together when you sat down, the tonus or resistance to stretch of those muscles will get progressively stronger as the muscles adaptively shorten to, and spend more time in, their new position.

Have you ever tried to stand up after sitting for a long time, whether at work or after a long car trip, and found that your body doesn't seem to want to let you stand up straight, but instead keeps you somewhat bent over? Although this usually passes after a short while as the muscles gradually release, what you experienced was your adaptively tightened hip flexor muscles holding you in a hip-flexed position. This is what happens when you spend a long time hip-flexed for any reason, and, although the tightness and bent-over posture usually go away pretty quickly, if this extended time in a hip-flexed position is repeated day after day, week after week, month after month, and year after year, eventually the muscles start to retain some of their adaptive shortening and don't return to their original resting length. When this happens, your pelvis begins to stay rotated forward, and the amount of the anterior rotation continues to increase over time with repeated, prolonged sitting unless something is done to correct it. Consequently, as we saw previously, when your pelvis tilts too far forward, it causes pain in your low back (and many other areas, which we'll discuss later), and because the root cause of this pain is adaptively shortened muscles from too much sitting even the best drugs and surgery won't address the root cause of the problem.

Obesity and pregnancy are two additional causes of an anteriorly rotated pelvis, and for the same reason. Instead of the body being in its normal proportion, both obesity and pregnancy involve the addition of a large amount of weight in the abdomen, out in front of the normal body outline, thereby changing the body's center of gravity and tilting the pelvis anteriorly. The same is true for women who are larger-breasted, as that involves a lot of extra weight in front of the chest. In all of these cases, the muscles in the back instinctively tighten to try to keep the body from falling forward, and when this tightening continues for a long time, as it does in all of these conditions, chronic pain in the back muscles usually isn't far behind (if you'll pardon the phrase).

Similarly, wearing high heels or cowboy boots is devastating to back muscles. Our legs are designed to be at roughly a 90-degree angle to the soles of our feet in a normal standing position. That means that if you put on raised heels that tilt the soles of your feet to, say, a 25-degree angle from the horizontal, your body would theoretically tilt forward 25 degrees from the vertical and you would fall on your face. Of course this doesn't happen, because your body is flexible and instinctively contracts a variety of back, neck, and leg muscles to try to keep you upright. Remember, however, that your body is contracting those muscles constantly, every minute that you're standing or walking in those raised heels, and as we've already seen, muscles in prolonged, constant contraction produce muscular tension and pain. Worse still, as if to add insult to injury, not only do the muscular contractions themselves cause pain, but many of the contracted muscles thereby strengthen their pull on the pelvis, rotating it still further anteriorly and causing more back pain, even after the offending footwear with the raised heels has been removed.

Because the best way to learn this is to experience it in your own body, try placing on the floor a book, catalog, or stack of magazines at least one inch thick, then stand in bare feet with your heels on the one inch lift and your toes on the floor. Relax for a moment and let your weight settle naturally on your feet. Now, keeping your entire upper body perfectly straight and rigid (like a soldier at attention), suddenly lock your knees straight. If you've done this correctly, you'll feel your upper body start to tilt forward and your toes and the balls of your feet will instinctively press down hard to keep you from falling forward, and you may even feel some of your back muscles start to tense up in an effort to keep you upright. Now try to repeat this test without pressing down with your feet or tightening your back muscles and you'll see that you'll fall on your face if you don't catch yourself. As you can see, wearing high heels causes the muscles in the legs and back to stay in constant contraction and hold your knees slightly flexed at all times just to keep you from falling over. If you want an even more powerful demonstration of this, try this test using a higher stack to simulate a two-inch or three-inch heel. Is it any wonder that wearing of high heels causes so much leg, back, and neck pain?

Nor is back pain the only consequence of an anteriorly rotated pelvis. When the pelvis rotates forward, the spine that sits on top of it rotates with it, so the body instinctively tries to correct for the resulting forward tilt of the spine. In addition to the low back muscles, the erector muscles that parallel the spine up the back and even as far as the skull all tighten to help bring the torso upright. Also, because the anterior rotation tends to make the neck incline forward, causing the face to tilt forward and down, the upper shoulder and posterior neck muscles that attach at the base of the back of the skull all tighten in order to rock the skull posteriorly so that the eyes can look straight ahead. This can result in headaches right there at the base of the skull, as well as headaches that spread along the side of the head over the ear and sometimes as far as the eye.

Even the eye muscles themselves get involved. There are muscles all around the outside of each eyeball to control its movement, and the muscles that attach on top of the eyeballs tighten when it's necessary to rotate the eyes upward. When an anterior pelvic rotation causes the face and the gaze to be turned somewhat downward toward the floor, these superior rectus muscles of the eyes instinctively tighten in an effort to help bring the gaze up to level. Although the posterior neck muscles do the bulk of the work by tilting the head back to make the gaze level, the superior rectus muscles also try to do their part, however small. When these eye muscles have to stay in constant contraction because of the anteriorly tilted pelvis and neck, they get fatigued and sore, just as any other muscles would, and can cause pain, headaches, and discomfort around the eyes.

Isn't that interesting? Did you realize that back pain, headaches, and eye pain could all result from something as simple and apparently innocuous as just sitting too much? Well, it's true, and now perhaps you can begin to see why standard treatments frequently don't work, or at least don't solve the problem permanently.

Well, you may be thinking, that's all well and good, but I don't have a choice: I have to sit all day to make my living, and I can't just quit my job. True enough, but there are things you can do to counteract the negative effects of habitual postures and help to keep yourself out of pain (as you'll see when we get to Section III).

Chapter 4

Pelvis Basics 2:
Tilting and Twisting to the Side

Although only in her early 50s, Donna felt that her life was over. A bright and vivacious woman who played competitive tennis at her country club, Donna had found herself in ever-increasing back, neck, and shoulder pain until she finally had to give up playing tennis. She had gone to a succession of doctors of all kinds who had run lots of inconclusive tests, but at best offered only sympathy and prescriptions for pain relief medication and at worst intimated that it might be all in her mind and offered to refer her to a psychiatrist. As she related this during our intake interview in my office, she broke down, saying, "I'm not crazy. I can't even get down on the floor to play with my grandchildren. Is this what it means to get old?"

After doing a thorough postural evaluation of Donna, I assured her that I absolutely did *not* think she was crazy. I explained that her pelvis was slightly smaller on the right side, causing her sacrum to tip down on the right and forcing the back, neck, and shoulder muscles on her left side to stay in constant contraction to keep her spine and head upright every minute that she was sitting or standing. Her tightly contracted muscles never got a moment's rest unless she was lying down; of course she was in pain!

I showed Donna how to put the correct thickness of material under the right side of her pelvis to level it when she was sitting and in her right shoe to level the pelvis when she was standing or walking. This let her back, neck, and shoulder muscles finally start to relax. Next, I suggested a program of home therapy, consisting of stretches, exercises, and movement therapy, all of which she did faithfully. Not only did her pain disappear, but before long she was back playing her beloved tennis.

Another distortion that I find in the vast majority of my clients is called a lateral pelvic tilt, in which one side of the pelvis is lower than the other, so that the pelvis tilts to either the right or left. The primary causes are anatomical leg length inequality (LLI), a small hemipelvis, and a fallen arch on one foot.

In my experience, the most common cause is anatomical leg length inequality, a condition in which the bones of one leg are simply shorter than those of the other leg. Although there are many possible causes for LLI, including injuries, surgeries, or disease, the most likely is probably genetics: That's just the way the bones grew. As noted in the previous chapter, we are not perfectly symmetrical beings, so it's always amazing to me when some writers on pain relief dismiss the frequency of LLI as being "statistically insignificant" or call LLI a "myth," because various studies have shown the prevalence of anatomical LLI ranging as high as 70 to 92 percent of people, although not everyone with LLI is symptomatic as a result. As an example, one study of 106 consecutive patients through a chiropractic clinic showed that 40 percent had a LLI of greater than 6 millimeters (about 1/4 inch) and that 70 percent had a LLI of greater than 3 millimeters (about 1/8 inch).[1]

In my practice, because I specialize in pain relief, I see a skewed sample of the population, because virtually everyone who sees me has some degree of pain, ranging from the slight to the disabling. Although I have never actually done a scientific survey of my records, I'd estimate that the percentage of people I see who have either a leg length inequality or a small hemipelvis is at least 95 percent and probably closer to 98 percent. In fact, if I measure someone and find both the legs and the two halves of the pelvis absolutely equal, I assume that I probably made a mistake and immediately retake those measurements a second or third time. Although there are occasional leg length differences of 1/2 inch or more, the vast majority of the leg length differences I find are in the 3/16- to 3/8-inch range, and the hemipelvis differences typically range from 1/8 inch to 3/16 inch.

If these differences sound insignificant, I can assure you they are not. Janet Travell, M.D., at one time the White House physician to President John F. Kennedy, and David G. Simons, M.D., co-authored a masterful two-volume medical text on muscles and the trigger points in them that cause pain. In discussing the various factors that can perpetuate pain, they say:

"The most common sources of such physical stress are skeletal asymmetry and disproportion. Asymmetries include a short leg—*a 0.5 cm (3/16 in) difference can be critical* [author's emphasis]—and a small hemipelvis."[2]

Later on, they add:

"To ensure lasting relief from the myofascial pain, it is important to correct a leg length discrepancy of as little as 0.3 cm (1/8 in) in a short person."[3]

Unfortunately, many physicians still regard anything less than an inch as not being a problem. When I discovered that I had about a 3/8-inch leg length difference and went to an orthopedic and spine clinic to get it X-rayed so my osteopath could measure the difference exactly on the film, the clinic doctor, an extremely experienced orthopedic specialist, told me, "Well, we'll go ahead and take a picture, but we really don't see much of a limp until it's at least an inch." Mind you, I wasn't there because of a limp; I was there because of raging, chronic back pain that had been tormenting me for almost 30 years, and that doctor's offhand dismissal of my condition as insignificant really angered me. Suffice it to say, once the 3/8-inch difference was confirmed and corrected for, my back pain just stopped. From the day I corrected my leg length difference by elevating the sole of my right shoe 3/8 inch, the back, hip, neck, and shoulder pain that had crippled me time and again for almost three decades quickly came to an end and from that day forward has never come back.

Nor am I the only one to have experienced this attitude on the part of the medical profession; many others have heard this, too. One of my clients went to her orthopedic physician at my request to have her legs and pelvis X-rayed and the differences measured exactly on the X-ray film, only to be told by the physician, not once but twice, that anything less than an inch wasn't really significant and that the body can compensate for smaller differences. Of course the body can and will instinctively compensate for the LLI by tightening certain muscles to try to pull the body upright and allow it to function better but, as we have already seen, that compensation means constant, prolonged contraction of those muscles, an extremely fertile source of musculoskeletal pain. As happens so often, when she experimented with self-correction of an apparent 3/16-inch difference, her life-altering pain disappeared and she was able once again to enjoy the sports and other activities she'd been forced to give up because of the pain.

To be fair, there are some physicians who recognize the importance of such apparently minor corrections, but in my experience they are few and far between. I was talking about this subject with one medical doctor who was also a chiropractor, and when I mentioned that my experience had shown the importance of correcting for even small leg length differences he replied, "Absolutely. I got rid of one patient's TMJ [jaw joint] pain just by putting a 1/8-inch lift in one of his shoes." Still, finding such a physician, one who recognizes the significance of these bone-length discrepancies in perpetuating pain and who regularly looks for and corrects them, is no easy matter, and you may have to kiss a lot of frogs before you find your Prince Charming.

Think of your legs as being two columns of bone that reach from the floor to your pelvis and on which your pelvis rests. Clearly, if one column of bone is shorter than the other, your pelvis will tilt to the shorter side, causing your spine to tilt the same way. However, because the spine is flexible, your body will instinctively try to curve it back to the opposite side so that your head and torso remain as upright and centered as possible, thus causing a scoliosis, a lateral curve in your spine. Naturally, this attempt by the Righting Reflex to keep you upright and balanced comes, as do most things in life, at a price, and in this case the price is constant muscular contraction every single minute you are on your feet, whether walking or standing. That muscular contraction can occur at several points along the spine, causing not only local pain in the involved muscles in the back and neck, but also referred pain into other parts of the body, including the head, face, chest, arm, hand, buttocks, and legs. This pain typically is worse when the sufferer has to stand for a prolonged period of time.

The LLI can occur in either the femur (thigh bone) or tibia (lower leg bone), or even in both, and this can usually be estimated fairly closely without an X-ray during a thorough postural evaluation by a trained evaluator. However, getting an exact measurement of any LLI requires an X-ray of the legs so that the bones can be measured on the X-ray film.

When I began to study leg length differences in detail, I noticed that some clients had suffered with the effects of LLI since childhood or their teenage years (as I had), yet others had only started to develop the symptoms much later in life, although the LLI had certainly existed at least since their bones had stopped growing in their late teenage years. Then, one day, after I had finished teaching a neuromuscular therapy seminar, I did a postural evaluation on my teaching assistant, who was almost precisely my height, my build, and my age, and who also, as it turned out, had the same 3/8-inch shorter right femur that I had. Knowing only too well the kind of pain such a difference can cause, I remarked, "You must have had a lot of back, hip, neck, or shoulder pain as a result of this LLI," to which he replied, "No, none; but you have to remember, I do a half-hour of stretching every morning of my life."

That was it: the answer to my puzzle. His muscles had to correct for the same amount of LLI as mine did, but his muscles, tendons, and ligaments were much more relaxed and limber, so his muscles didn't have to contract as hard as mine did to compensate for the tilt caused by the shorter leg. When people are either naturally limber or do a lot of stretching to make themselves so, the LLI may cause little or no pain for many years, but as those people age and the elasticity of their muscles, tendons, and ligaments tends to decrease, their muscles now have to contract harder against the increased resistance and nagging musculoskeletal pain begins to appear as if out of nowhere.

In addition to leg length inequality, the other major skeletal asymmetry that can create a tilted pelvis is a condition called a small hemipelvis. If you look back at Figure 2-1, you'll see that the pelvis has two halves, each of which is called a hemipelvis (also known anatomically as the innominate bone), one on either side of the sacrum. Just as one leg can be shorter than the other, one hemipelvis can be smaller than the other, although in my experience a small hemipelvis is not quite as common as a leg length inequality. However, when a small hemipelvis exists, the top surface of the sacrum typically tilts down slightly on the side of the smaller hemipelvis, thereby causing the spine to tilt to one side as it arises from the tilted sacrum, just as in the case of a shorter leg, and this tilt likewise causes the Righting Reflex to tighten muscles and create a scoliosis, a lateral or sideways curvature of the spine, in an effort to try to keep the head and torso as upright as possible. Once again, we're back to constant muscular contraction and the consequent pain it causes.

Let's digress for a moment to discuss scoliosis. Although there are many causes listed for scoliosis in medical textbooks, one thing is certain: If the top of the sacrum is tilted, the spinal column that arises from it will be tilted, and, in its instinctive attempt to correct that tilt and bring the eyes level with the horizon, the Righting Reflex will curve the spine and create a scoliosis. Put simply, a lateral pelvic tilt *must* create a scoliosis, except in two rare cases:

1. Where a vertebra immediately above the sacrum is misshapen in such a way that it tilts to the opposite side to the same degree, thus making its top surface level.

2. Where the sacrum itself is misaligned within the pelvis so that it tilts to the opposite side to the same degree, likewise making its top surface level.

That's why it's helpful to have children evaluated for leg length and pelvic asymmetries early in life, because that will allow for early correction of any asymmetries found and help to minimize, or perhaps even avert, later problems with scoliosis. (We'll talk more about this issue later.)

Unfortunately, a small hemipelvis has a greater potential for causing pain than does a LLI, although a LLI can sometimes cause severe, life-altering pain. Remember that we said that a LLI causes your compensating muscles to remain contracted every minute that you're standing or walking; usually, however, you can get some temporary relief by sitting down, because your unequal legs are no longer supporting you and you can sit upright naturally on your pelvis without tilting. With a small hemipelvis, though, the two halves of the pelvis itself are unequal, one smaller than the other, so that when you sit down, your whole body still tilts toward the side with the smaller hemipelvis. Consequently, if you have a small hemipelvis, you get no relief from your standing pain by sitting down, because the distortion still exists in the sitting position and the compensating muscles still have to maintain their constant contraction; the only way you'll get relief is by lying down so that the muscles won't have to support the tilting spine against gravity and can finally relax. People with this condition typically find it difficult to sit comfortably for very long, often shifting their positions repeatedly, and frequently feeling as though they are leaning to one side a little when they sit. They often describe themselves as "restless," and this restlessness could be mistaken as a sign of hyperactivity. Fortunately, however, there is a simple way to correct for a small hemipelvis and bring amazing relief to many sufferers, as we'll see in Section III when we address solutions for the various problems we're outlining.

As mentioned, a collapsed medial longitudinal arch in one foot can cause an apparent or functional leg length difference, even though the legs may be anatomically equal in length. Let's assume that your left foot has a normal medial longitudinal arch (the arch that runs from the front of your heel to the ball of your big toe), but that the arch under your right foot has fallen or collapsed. This will cause your right foot to tilt and collapse inward, toward the inside of the foot, and as it does so the entire right leg drops with it. Consequently, even though the actual bone lengths of the two legs may be absolutely equal, the top of the right leg, where it supports the pelvis, will have dropped so that it is lower than the top of the left leg, thereby causing the pelvis to tilt downward on the right.

Please note, though, that this *does* not apply to everybody with fallen or dropped arches in their feet. It only applies if *one* of the arches is dropped and the other is not. If both arches are equal—whether both collapsed, both normal, or both high—the effect on the two sides will be equal and, assuming the anatomical bone lengths of the legs are equal, the tops of the legs should be at the same height and the pelvis should be level.

Finally, there is the question of whether tight muscles on one side of the pelvis, between the top of the pelvis and the top of the femur or thigh bone, could perhaps tend to pull the top edge of the pelvis down, causing a pelvic tilt to the tight side. Because a normal pelvis is a strongly ligamented bony framework, not easily distorted by muscular contraction, a downward pull on, say, the left side of the pelvis would cause the left side of the pelvis to rotate around the head of the left femur at the hip joint, thereby forcing the right side of the pelvis to rise. However, because the right side of the pelvis is firmly attached to the right leg at the hip joint, this would require the right side of the pelvis to lift the right leg off the ground and hold it there while standing, which, even if it could occur, would make any standing leg length evaluation meaningless by definition. In my experience, except in those cases where distortion occurs within the pelvis, tight lateral pelvic muscles are not a cause of lateral pelvic tilt, although I almost always find these muscles tight as an effect of one of the other causes. I have found that far and away the most common causes are anatomical leg length inequality, a small hemipelvis, or a collapsed arch in one foot, and these are fortunately relatively easy to remedy (as we'll discover in Section III).

In addition to the pain caused by the tight muscles involved in both the lateral pelvic tilt and the resulting postural compensations, the downward tilt of the ribcage on the low shoulder side puts pressure on the organs found on that side, and even more so if the low shoulder and the high side of the pelvis occur on the same side. For example, if the pelvis is tilted high right and the shoulder is tilted low right, sharply narrowing the space between the right shoulder and pelvis, not only will the muscles of the right side be adaptively shortened and tender but the liver and gall bladder, which are located in the upper right abdomen, will be compressed as well. If the reverse occurs, with a high left pelvis and low left shoulder, organs in the upper left abdomen—the stomach, spleen, and pancreas—will be compressed. Obviously, an organ that is compressed can hardly be expected to function as well as one that has its own natural free space, and the long-term compression of organs can potentially have a significant deleterious effect on their health and function.

This kind of compression also occurs when we stand or sit with a forward-collapsing, slumping posture. Sit perfectly erect for a moment and hook the tips of your fingers under the lower edge of the front of your rib cage; now let yourself slump forward. Did you feel how the edge of the rib cage collapsed downward and slightly inward? When it does so, it puts pressure on many of the digestive organs, including the stomach, transverse colon, and small intestine, as well as on the liver, gall bladder, and pancreas.

This collapsed posture also affects the lungs and diaphragm, making breathing more difficult. To experience this, slump forward again, as you just did. Now, while keeping that slumped posture, try to take a deep breath. Tough to do, isn't it? That's why people who habitually sit and/or stand with a slumped posture tend to have shallow breathing, resulting in diminished oxygen intake, along with a consequent lack of energy and reduced oxygenation of the muscles, with the latter in turn contributing to increased muscular tension and pain throughout the body.

Nor is this all. Compression from postural distortion also affects the acupuncture meridians that run throughout the body. When this kind of compression occurs, the flow of "chi" or vital energy through the meridians in that area is blocked, causing what acupuncturists call stagnation. Stagnation of chi can cause diminished vitality and reduced energy and, if the stagnation persists for a long time, can result in organ dysfunction. It's hardly any wonder, then, that people with chronic slumping postures or other major postural distortions often have major problems with digestion, breathing, and lack of energy.

Rotational Distortions

Last, but not least, in our examination of the pelvis, let's look at rotational distortions. Rotational distortions occur when some part of the body at rest, either standing or lying down, is twisted to the right or left. As an example, let's take a case where the right side of the pelvis and the right shoulder are anterior (forward) when compared with the corresponding parts on the left side of the body. This creates a lateral rotation of the body to the left, with several negative consequences.

To understand it better, try feeling the effects in your own body. Stand with the backs of your heels up against a line in the floor or the carpet, or else put a magazine, board, or other straight-edged item on the floor and back up until the backs of your heels are up against the edge of it so that the heels of the two feet are even (that is, neither foot is in front of the other). This ensures that you don't start out with a natural rotation, because if, for example, you stand with your right foot slightly forward of the left, your torso will, of course, rotate to the left.

With your heels now even, and keeping your feet in place, turn your body so that the right side of your pelvis is forward of the left by a couple of inches. (Although this is a little more of a rotation than is usually found, exaggerating it slightly helps you to feel the effects more readily while you're learning.) You'll notice that your trunk and shoulders tend naturally to turn to the left with your pelvis and that your head tends to turn left also to keep you looking in the same direction that your chest is facing.

The problem with this position, though, is that although your feet are pointing straight ahead, say toward the 12 on an imaginary clock dial on the floor, your eyes and chest are facing the 10 or 11. As you'll readily appreciate, it's both difficult and potentially dangerous to be walking in one direction and looking in another, so your body instinctively turns your head back around to face the direction your feet are going, toward the 12. If you keep your torso turned to the left while turning your head to face forward (toward the 12), you'll notice that this position tends to tighten several of the muscles of the neck. This muscle tension might not seem all that much now, but imagine keeping that twist in your neck constantly throughout the day. Those muscles are required to stay in a state of constant contraction to keep you looking where you're going and, as you already know by now, muscles in a prolonged state of constant contraction are a recipe for pain. Your body is turning to the left, your head is compensating by turning right so you can see straight ahead, and your neck is being twisted like a dishrag being wrung out.

Sometimes, though, this twist occurs not in the neck, but in the middle of the back. Stand as you did before, with your heels even and the right side of your pelvis forward, but instead of letting your right shoulder go forward too, turn your left shoulder forward instead. Remember not to let your pelvis change position; you want the right side of your pelvis and the left shoulder both to be forward. In this case, with your pelvis turning left and your shoulders turning right, it's the middle of your back that's being wrung out like a dishrag. Pretty uncomfortable, isn't it?

Nor is this all. In the position just described, if your pelvis stays forward on the right and your left shoulder comes forward enough so that it's more forward than the right shoulder, not only will you have the "dishrag effect" in the middle of your back, but in your neck as well, because your head will now have to turn back to the left to face in the direction your feet are pointing. Not only do these counter-rotations that produce this "dishrag effect" involve the constant contraction of numerous muscles, they also cause the vertebrae in the spine to twist with respect to their adjacent vertebrae, as well as compressing the vertebrae together. These twisting and compression forces are transmitted to the intervertebral disks and tend over time to break down the disks and flatten them.

If you're wondering how many people really have these rotational distortions, the answer, in my experience, is most people. I see these kinds of rotations in my practice on a daily basis and, although the majority of the rotational distortions are not dramatic, the constant muscular contraction and disk compression involved can contribute significantly to a person's burden of chronic pain and fatigue.

Chapter 5

Other Distortions:
Paying the Penalty of Our Modern Lifestyle

A computer professional himself, Bob had experienced the arm, hand, neck, and head pain that comes from extended computer use, but the story he told me as I worked on his forearms really made me think. He had been sitting in a friend's living room when his friend's 9-year-old daughter came in from her bedroom complaining of arm and hand pain from using the mouse to play computer games. I couldn't help wondering what kind of pain this little girl would be experiencing at her high school graduation after nine more years of ever more intensive computer use, not to mention after four years of college, before she even started her career in a computer-driven world.

Shoulder and neck distortions can occur either on their own or as a result of pelvic distortions down below. As we have already seen, when a pelvis tilts for any reason, the Righting Reflex causes the spine to curve in order to try to keep us as upright and functional as possible. This spinal compensation continues right on up into the neck, causing neck muscles to tighten and thereby creating pain.

Let's take a case where the pelvis is low on one side. If the right side of the pelvis is lower, you might reasonably assume that the right shoulder would be lower, too, but this is not always the case. Sometimes, for any one of a number of reasons, such as habitual postural distortion while working or perhaps an unresolved muscular compensation for an old injury, the shoulders tilt in the opposite direction, so that the left hip is high and the left shoulder is low.

In either case, any time your shoulders tilt to one side, the muscles that run along your high shoulder and up the back of your neck will usually be tighter and more tender than the corresponding muscles on your low side. Why? Well, remember that bones are supposed to carry weight, whereas muscles are only designed to move bones. When the shoulders tilt, the head naturally tends to tilt to the low side, but the Righting Reflex tries to keep the eyes level with the horizon, so the high side shoulder muscles contract to pull the head erect and level the eyes. Because those muscles have to maintain constant contraction every moment you're upright in order to prevent the head from tilting back to the low side, they naturally become tight and painful.

Another extremely common source of pain is anteriorly rotated shoulders, in which the shoulders, instead of being directly to either side of the body, are actually pulled forward around the body. This is most often caused by spending lots of time with our hands in front of us, as most of us do when working (such as writing at a desk, typing at a computer, or driving) and even in our leisuretime activities. Whether you are an attorney, auto mechanic, billing clerk, surgeon, truck driver, or pianist, if you spend any significant amount of time with your hands in front of you, the pectoralis muscles of your chest adaptively shorten and pull your shoulders forward, until finally they are actually holding your shoulders forward even when your arms are at rest at your sides.

If you look again at the front view in Figure 2-1, you'll see that the hands are at the sides with the backs of the hands facing outward directly to the left and right and that you can see through the space between the thumb and fingers on each side. To see how you compare, stand in front of a full length mirror, close your eyes, wiggle your shoulders and arms around briefly so that they stay loose and natural, then let your shoulders settle into whatever position feels natural. Remember: Don't try to pose in any particular position; just stand as you normally stand. Now open your eyes. Note where your hands are. If they're positioned as those in the front view in the illustration are, congratulations! If, however, you notice that your hands are actually forward, especially if they are starting to come around toward the front of the thigh, your shoulders are rotated anteriorly. To see what erect posture feels like, gently pull your shoulder blades together until your elbows come back around to the sides of your body, just above where the stripe on the side of a pair of uniform pants would be. After you've held this for a while, release the muscular contraction between your shoulder blades and let your shoulders relax. Now, as your shoulders move into their "normal" posture, you can feel (and see in the mirror) how anterior shoulder rotation affects your body.

Another way to determine if your shoulders are anteriorly rotated is to notice how your arms swing when you walk. With good posture, our arms should swing at our sides exactly parallel to our line of motion; if, however, we notice that our hands tend to swing across in front of our body slightly, that's a sign that our shoulders are pulled anteriorly. Think of yourself for a moment as a little wooden soldier with wooden arms that are each held on with a single nail and swing freely on those nails. If the nails are driven straight into each side of the upper body, the arms will swing exactly parallel to your line of march. If, however, we were to bend those nails forward on each side, the arms would now swing somewhat in front of the body every time they come forward, then out and away from the body as they swing back.

Okay, so your shoulders are somewhat anteriorly rotated; how does that affect you? Profoundly, and in several ways. First of all, when your shoulders come forward, your neck tends to incline forward, too. When the shoulders are anterior, the neck and head are typically pulled forward into what's called a forward head posture, where the ear (in side view), instead of being properly aligned above the center of the shoulder (see Figure 2-1, side view), is instead somewhat forward of the shoulder. Think of a bowling ball sitting on the top of a fence post. As long as the fence post is vertical, the bowling ball sits there just fine, but if the post is tilted forward, the weight of the ball tends to make it fall forward. Similarly, when your shoulders rotate anteriorly, your neck generally tilts forward, too, which in turn would cause your head to fall forward, were it not for the muscles in the back of your neck, which are then forced into constant contraction to hold your head up. Remember that muscles are not designed to contract constantly, so the result will be pain and dysfunction.

You can also think of it this way. Because your neck and head tend to tilt forward as your shoulders are pulled anteriorly, that causes your gaze to tilt forward, too, with the result that you'd end up looking down slightly as you are walking along or sitting at your computer. However, because you need to see where you're walking or what you're doing on the computer monitor, you have to bring your gaze up, which your body does instinctively by tightening the muscles at the base of your skull in the back, right at the top of your neck, and along the tops of your shoulders. Not only do these posterior neck and shoulder muscles themselves get tight and painful, but they frequently form trigger points that refer pain all along the sides of the head and into the temples, ears, and eyes. When you add to this the trigger points in the adaptively shortened muscles in the sides of your neck that refer pain into the forehead, eyes, ears, jaw, face, and neck, is it any wonder that headaches and neck and shoulder pain are so common?

Anteriorly rotated shoulders can also be a cause of upper back pain. When your shoulders get pulled around in front as your chest muscles shorten and tighten, the back muscles between your shoulder blades get stretched horizontally, which can cause them to ache. Likewise, as your head and neck come forward, the erector muscles that run up the back along your spine also get stretched vertically and can become painful. Because these conditions tend to occur together, your upper/middle back gets a double whammy, because the muscles there are stretched both vertically and horizontally, with the common center of the two stretches typically located roughly between the shoulder blades. Is it any wonder that our backs ache when we sit or stand for long periods with our shoulders rolled forward?

Do any of those neck, shoulder, back, or headache symptoms sound familiar? Because the nature of our modern society is such that many of us spend many hours each day with our hands in front of us, and because we repeat this postural pattern every work day for weeks, months, and even years on end, these pain complaints are incredibly widespread, and numbing them with pain relievers doesn't resolve the problem. Only by finding the root cause of the problem and restoring postural integrity can the pain ever go away for good.

In addition to tight chest muscles pulling the shoulders forward, there are several other common causes of anterior shoulder rotation and the consequent forward head posture. Sitting, standing, or walking in a slumped posture tilts the shoulders forward, naturally causing the neck and head to fall forward and thereby starting the same chain of consequences previously described. Likewise, if the pelvis is anteriorly rotated (tilted forward), the top of the sacrum is tilted forward, which in turn causes the rest of the spine to arise from the sacrum in an anteriorly tilted position. This tends to throw the shoulders forward, as well as causes the erector muscles along the spine to tighten constantly in order to counteract the anterior pelvic rotation and try to hold the torso upright. Similarly, when the pelvis is rotated posteriorly (tilted backward), forcing the sacrum—and therefore the spine—to tilt backward and shift the body's center of gravity posteriorly, the head and shoulders instinctively move forward to counterbalance that shift and keep the center of gravity safely forward, within its normal range.

Nor is this all the harm that results from anteriorly rotated shoulders. When the shoulders are pulled forward by tight chest muscles, those tight muscles can restrict the full expansion of the lungs, thereby restricting breathing. This not only saps and limits our energy but can adversely affect the oxygenation of the body's muscles, thereby contributing to pain. Many times, after I've released the tension in someone's chest muscles, I've heard the comment, "I can breathe better now." Furthermore, if the anteriorly rotated shoulders are combined with the collapsed, slumping posture we discussed in the last chapter, the downward and inward pressure of the lower edge of the ribcage puts pressure directly onto several internal structures, including the stomach, transverse colon, diaphragm, liver, gall bladder, and pancreas. How often, though, is poor posture considered and treated as a significant contributor to organ disease and dysfunction?

As for arm distortions, we use our arms and hands in almost everything we do, so it's hardly surprising that they often develop painful spots and trigger points in their muscles as a result of either habitual posture or overuse, or both. We've already seen how anteriorly rotated shoulders can cause the arms to move forward so that the hands start to hang more toward the front of the thighs than by the sides. There are several possible arm distortions, but in my experience the most common by far is called pronation of the forearms. If your shoulders are back where they belong and you bend your elbows to a right angle while keeping your upper arms at your sides, your forearms should be sticking out in front of you on either side with the palms facing each other, thumbs uppermost. This is a normal, neutral hand position. Now turn your palms down, as if in position to type on a computer, write at a desk, or play the piano; this position is called pronation, meaning that the forearms and hands have turned prone, or face down.

Although occasional pronation isn't a problem, a lot of people in today's society spend a tremendous amount of time with their forearms pronated, often for hours on end, and especially when working at computers, both on the keyboard and the mouse. Because the normal position of the hands in front of us is that neutral, thumbs up position, it takes constant contraction of the pronator muscles to hold the hands in position to type on a keyboard, use a computer mouse, write a letter, or play the piano. As a result, after many days, weeks, months, or years of holding our hands in that unnatural position, it's not surprising that we may suddenly become aware that our forearms remain pronated when they hang at our sides, with the backs of our hands tending to face forward, rather than out to the sides.

I've found forearm pronation to be extremely common, in varying degrees, among people who work a great deal at computers, as are the forearm, wrist, and hand tension and pain that so frequently accompany it. That tension and pain are the results not just of the constantly contracted pronator muscles, although they certainly contribute their share, but of all the muscles that are kept in almost constant contraction in order to hold the arms, wrists, and hands in that unnatural position for long periods of time.

Lest you think that this problem is just confined to a few computer geeks who have been working 60-hour weeks on computers for the last 10 years, remember the example at the beginning of this chapter of the 9-year-old girl with pain in her arm and hand from playing computer games. With children now beginning to use computers earlier and earlier in life (practically before the children are weaned!), this intense overuse and postural distortion has the potential to create pain problems for an ever-growing number of people, and even at very young ages. Fortunately, there are ways to help counteract these effects of prolonged computer use (as you'll see in Section III).

Postural Distortion Summary

In Chapter 3, we talked about the three possible distortions at the pelvis: side to side tilt, anterior or posterior rotation, and rotation left or right (see Figure 3-1). As I also noted, the great majority of the people I've measured have all three of these distortions to some extent, along with the upper body distortions that result when the pelvis isn't properly aligned.

Even if you have all three pelvic distortions, it's probably difficult, if not impossible, for you to feel their effects in your body because over many years your brain has already accepted these distortions as "normal." If you want to feel what it's like to have all three distortions, you need to exaggerate or increase each one slightly.

Let's take a combined pattern that I see frequently. Begin by putting a thick magazine or thin book (perhaps 1/2-inch thick) on the floor, then stand with your left foot on the book and your right foot on the floor. Let your weight settle into this new position and really pay attention to your muscles, noting especially where they feel as though they're tightening. Now add an anterior pelvic tilt, rocking the top of your pelvis forward and holding it there by contracting the quadriceps muscles in the front of your thighs. Don't forget, though, that although this will tilt your whole torso forward, you can't go through life tilted forward like that, so while keeping your pelvis tilted forward, try to pull your spine erect. Feel that ache in your back as those muscles contract? Finally, while holding all the distortions you've created so far, twist the right side of your pelvis and your right shoulder forward and around toward the left, then turn your head back toward the right so you can face forward (the direction your feet are facing). If you've done all this according to the directions, you should be pretty uncomfortable about now. This gives you an experience in your own body of the pain that postural distortion can cause.

Now stand normally, step off the magazine or book, and do some stretching and movement to relax the muscles you just contracted. Not much fun, was it? Yet that sort of musculoskeletal pain, to a greater or lesser degree, is the daily companion to millions of people the world over. It ranges from the nagging aches that just never seem to go away to disabling pain that distorts bodies and ruins lives. Pain relievers and muscle-relaxing drugs certainly have a valuable place in medicine but, if your pain or muscle spasm is due to an anatomical leg length inequality, a tilted or rotated pelvis, or anteriorly rotated shoulders and a forward head posture, these medications will only mask the symptoms, leaving the root cause of your pain untouched. Only when the underlying postural distortions are corrected will the muscles finally be able to relax and the pain diminish for good.

Some causes of pain are strictly anatomical in nature, such as a leg length inequality, a small hemipelvis, or a collapsed arch in one foot, and because these relate to our structural foundation it is imperative to correct for these skeletal asymmetries before beginning other corrective measures, as otherwise the body will continue to experience the pain that comes with standing or sitting on a tilted foundation. Other causes of pain are simply the penalties of our modern lifestyle, the habitual postures we assume in the course of our daily work or other activities. Except in rare and very severe circumstances it's not necessary to quit our jobs in order to get well, but it *is* necessary to counterbalance the effects of our habitual postures and actions if we want to remain pain-free.

Although I help people to make these kinds of corrections every day in my office by releasing their tight muscles, only they can tighten their loose muscles, and besides, there aren't enough therapists in the world to treat even a fraction of the people with musculoskeletal pain. Fortunately, there are ways that you can get and keep yourself out of pain, or else keep yourself from developing pain in the first place, and these are the things I try to teach my clients. That's what the rest of this book is about.

Now that you've mastered the basics, let's take a look at your posture.

Section II

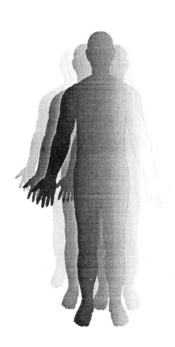

Charting Your Posture

Chapter 6

Posture-Charting Basics:
Getting Ready

Carol always dressed stylishly, loved to wear nice clothes, and looked great in them, but she was frustrated because she always had to have the right leg of her slacks or the right side of her dress hemmed up so the two sides would look even. She also had chronic hip, neck, and back pain (although she was probably more distressed by her tailoring problems!). When a postural evaluation showed that she had a short right femur, not only did a 1/4-inch elevation in her right shoe level her pelvis and get rid of the majority of her chronic pain, it also resolved her hem line problem.

If you've ever looked in the mirror and noticed that one shoulder seemed to be higher than the other, or if you've discovered that you need to have the legs of your pants hemmed to different lengths, you've already entered the world of postural analysis. The toughest, yet most important, part of this whole process is getting an accurate evaluation of your posture; once you know what your postural distortions are, correcting them is a pretty logical and straightforward process. Although it usually takes less than 15 minutes for a trained evaluator to do a basic postural analysis, there are nowhere near enough trained evaluators to help the tens of millions of people in pain in this country and around the world. Until that day comes, my hope is that by showing you how to look at your own posture and use simple stretches and exercises to correct the distortions you find, I can help you to learn how to free yourself from musculoskeletal pain and to keep yourself pain-free. Various healing professions look at the structure of the body in different ways and do different types of postural evaluations, but the simplified approach you're about to learn will give you a clear picture of your posture and make it easy to see the areas where changes are needed.

Three things have to be borne in mind as you begin this process. First, there is no way you can do a meaningful postural evaluation on yourself, because you can't reach to measure, twist to look, and still stand in your usual relaxed posture. Although you may be able to see a few things accurately on your own in the mirror, it takes a second person or partner to be able to get worthwhile results on most of the measurements, so you and a partner will take turns measuring each other.

Second, the method you'll learn in this book is only an abbreviated version of a much more comprehensive evaluation I do in my office, one that I evolved originally from a method generally used by St. John neuromuscular therapists. Unless you have considerable knowledge of musculoskeletal anatomy, a number of the more involved measurement techniques would be difficult to teach, especially in a book rather than in person. This abbreviated version will "cut to the chase" and give you just the basic techniques necessary to get enough information to be able to successfully plan your postural corrections in most cases.

Third, there are many borderline or complex cases for which this method will be inappropriate or insufficient. In those cases, it is strongly recommended that you get your posture evaluated by a properly trained professional.

The basic idea of postural analysis is simple and logical. We saw in Section I that in ideal posture the body is aligned on the midsagittal, coronal, and horizontal planes (see Figure 2-1), and we've also seen from our discussion so far that, when the body deviates from this ideal posture, muscles chronically tighten, thereby causing pain. Consequently, a postural analysis is done to determine how a particular body is deviating from ideal postural alignment so that we can find and correct the muscular imbalances that cause pain. By determining what postural discrepancies exist—if one hip is higher than the other, if one shoulder is forward of the other, and so forth—we can draw a "map" of the body as it is. Once we have drawn and understand that "map," we can directly chart our way out of pain.

Think of it this way: If we drive into a town we've never been to before and we're trying to find a certain address, we can drive all over town randomly, hoping to come across that address by dumb luck, but that wastes time and money, as well as being incredibly inefficient and foolish. If, however, we first obtain a map of this heretofore unknown town, we can quickly and easily drive directly to our goal. Similarly, in trying to solve a musculoskeletal pain problem, before rushing off in all directions to try this or that therapy, or to do some indiscriminate stretching and exercise, it makes far more sense first to analyze the musculoskeletal structure as it is so that we can figure out how to reach our postural goals intelligently and effectively and thereby get ourselves out of pain.

Procedure for Evaluation

Although you can start your postural evaluation with any part of the body, I find it both logical and effective to begin with the feet, as they form the foundation of the body. After that, I continue to measure points up the front of the body, then down the back, after which I check the person from both sides. In my clinic, I also check several points with the person lying on my treatment table, but that won't be necessary for the purposes of this book. To record your findings, feel free to copy the postural evaluation form shown in Figure 2-1 and mark it up as necessary. (**NOTE: Although this book is copyrighted, and copying copyrighted works is illegal without permission, this is your permission to copy that one illustration, Figure 2-1, as needed for your personal, noncommercial use.**) I suggest using a pencil with a good eraser, as even the most experienced therapist can make mistakes, and being able to erase incorrect or unwanted lines makes the chart much easier to read.

Note also that the directions given are for you, as the evaluator, to measure your partner. When you've done all the measurements and properly recorded them on your partner's chart, simply trade places and have your partner measure you.

Dress

The person being evaluated should wear minimal clothing, consistent with modesty, and should be in bare feet, although shoes should be kept handy, as they may be required in the course of the evaluation in some circumstances. In my office, I suggest that people wear either light workout clothes (for example, running shorts for men, running shorts and a sports bra for women) or bathing suits. Shorts made of a heavy material, such as denim, are not desirable, as they have bulky seams and dense fabric that make it difficult to feel some of the points you're going to measure, so shorts made of a light fabric are best. Shirts cover up a lot of the points you'll want to measure, and although an experienced therapist can do a postural evaluation right through a shirt and pants, you'll find that while you're learning it's a lot easier to measure someone if you can see what you're measuring. Don't get caught up in issues of fashion here; all that's needed is light, minimal clothing that will allow you to easily see or feel the bony landmarks you'll be looking for.

Positioning

To begin the evaluation, have your partner stand facing you in his or her normal posture. Be sure not to give any specific instructions on how to stand, other than perhaps something along the lines of "stand naturally" or "just be yourself." The idea is not to have your partner stand in any particular posture at this point, but rather to see how he or she naturally stands. If your partner seems a bit stiff or posed, have him or her step up and down in place a few times and perhaps shake the shoulders up and down and back and forth a few times, then let the body settle out as it will. This often helps to relax someone who is self-conscious or is actively trying to maintain "good" posture. Remember: You don't want to measure your partner's idea of "good" posture; you want to measure your partner's normal, everyday posture, because it's the everyday posture that helps produce the everyday pain.

Important Points to Remember

A few suggestions are in order here, and they apply to all the measurements you'll be taking. First of all, you must get your eyes directly in front of what you're measuring and (other than when measuring the arches) precisely at the level of the measurement; otherwise, angular distortion will almost certainly cause you to see the measurement incorrectly. This may require that you bend your knees or kneel in order to get your eyes where they need to be, but if you want to get meaningful results, there's no other way. I try to think of it as good exercise that helps to keep me young!

Second, there's a common tendency to try subconsciously to make measurements come out the way we expect them to. If you think someone has a high right shoulder, there's often a tendency to subconsciously position your hands so that, sure enough, the right shoulder does appear higher. You can avoid this by locating the bony landmarks that you're trying to measure, getting your hands approximately into position, then looking away from your hands while you concentrate on positioning your hands properly and noticing whether your hands feel as though they're in the same place on both sides of the body. Once your hands feel as though they're in the right position and you're ready to take the measurement, simply turn your head to look at your hands and quickly note what you see. By looking away as you get into position, then suddenly looking back and taking your reading, you have a better chance of seeing the measurement as it really is and you don't give yourself a chance to "create" the measurement you expect.

Third, please don't agonize over trying to detect minute differences; you're looking for differences that, whether larger or smaller, are clearly discernible. Also, please remember that it's okay for a measurement to be level or equal on both sides! All too often in classes I've seen students struggling desperately to determine, for example, which side of the pelvis is higher, on the assumption that they must be missing something if they can't see a difference between the two sides. If you're not sure of your first measurement, by all means take a second measurement, or even a third if need be; if I'm not sure of a measurement, I'll remeasure it as many times as I need to until I think I have it right. Remember the old carpenter's motto, "Measure twice, saw once"; it's always a good idea to double check to make sure you've gotten your measurements right before you start your work, because it can save you from having to redo it later. However, if you get the same measurement two or three times, mark it accordingly and trust it for now. If subsequent measurement or other information causes you to change your mind, you can always change your marking on the chart. Learn to trust your measurements, and have fun!

Finally, please remember that even the most apparently exact measurements you take are still likely to be at best an approximation. Although an experienced evaluator, after doing literally hundreds of postural evaluations using this system, can be surprisingly accurate the vast majority of the time, even then the possibility of error is ever present. In some cases, only an X-ray can determine the postural truth, so don't get down on yourself if subsequent evaluation indicates that your initial measurements were off slightly, and remember that if you carefully follow the instructions given in Section III (on Getting Rid of Your Pain), you won't do any harm even if one of your measurements turns out to be slightly incorrect.

Ready? Let's start measuring.

Chapter 7

A Keen Eye, Part 1:
Measuring From the Front

An avid ski racer, Nick was plagued with hip and low back pain that he attributed to the intense days he spent on the slopes. Having noticed in the course of the postural evaluation that his right hip was projected forward, I asked him as I was working on his back muscles if his ski turns to the left were easier to do than those to the right. His head spun around to look up at me and he said, "My coach is always yelling at me because my turns are different. How'd you know that?" I explained that, because his right hip was forward, turning his pelvis to the left, his body was already turning left, making left turns easy and natural, whereas turning to the right was going "against the grain," against the twist of his body, making right turns more difficult. Once he understood that this twist was due to an imbalance in the muscles of his pelvis and upper legs, he was more than eager to do the corrective stretches and exercises I gave him as homework to realign his pelvis. Not only did his ski turns improve, so did his hip and back pain.

Feet

First of all, look at the way the feet are pointing. If they point essentially straight ahead, that's great; just mark them with arrows as shown in Figure 7-1a. If one or both feet turn out or in, you can use arrows to indicate that, as shown in Figure 7-1b and Figure 7-1c.

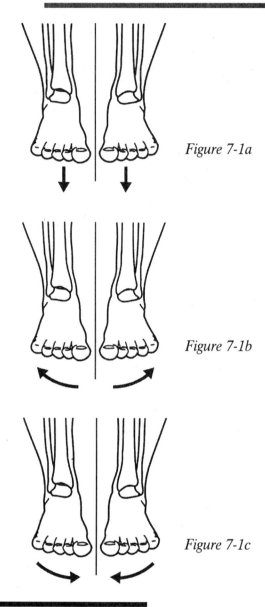

Figure 7-1a

Figure 7-1b

Figure 7-1c

Figure 7-1

Next, it's time to check the arches. For this measurement, make sure that the feet are at least four or five inches apart before proceeding. To see how high or low the arches are, place your right index finger, nail side down, on the floor between the feet and pointing toward the inside of the right foot. Gently insert your index finger under the right foot, approximately in the middle of the arch. For a rough guide to locate the middle of the arch, envision an imaginary line down the front of the shin that continues along the inside of the foot to the ground. Where that line touches the ground is about where you want to take your measurement (see Figure 7-2a).

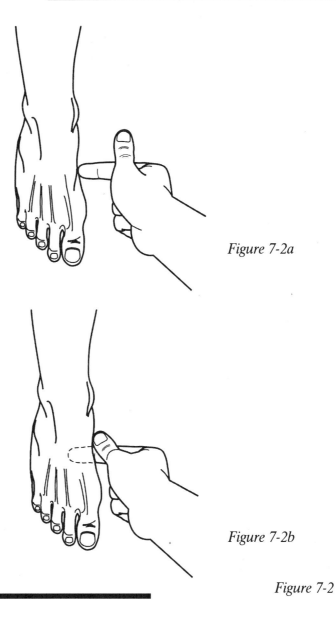

Figure 7-2a

Figure 7-2b

Figure 7-2

As you gently stick your index finger under the arch, only go under far enough to meet the resistance of the skin; never force your way under. Next, leaving your right index finger under the arch, bring the edge of your right thumb up against the inside of the foot, then press it down against your finger to act as a marker to show how far the thumb went under (see Figure 7-2b). Now, keeping your thumb and finger pressed together, pull your finger tip out from under the arch and repeat the process with your left index finger under your partner's left arch.

Now, look at how much of your finger is sticking out past the edge of your thumb on each hand. As a rough guide, if your index finger went under the arch all the way up to about the first joint, the arch is probably pretty good. By contrast, if the arch has totally collapsed, you won't even be able to get your finger under the arch at all. Most arches will usually be somewhere in between these two measurements.

To record these measurements on the chart, look at the examples in Figure 7-3. Figure 7-3a shows the chart marked with a line slanted down toward the midline of the body as a means of indicating that the arch has collapsed inward. Figure 7-3b shows the line slanted down toward the outside of the body to indicate that the arch is extremely high and the feet are rocked outward onto their outside edges. If the arches appear normal, either draw the lines straight across at each ankle or else just mark an "X" on the end of each line to indicate that you checked them and that they were "x-actly" where they should be. Some people like to try to give their slanted lines more or less slant to indicate how much the arch has dropped or elevated, or to indicate the severity of any measured distortion, but it's difficult to remember later on what a given degree of line slant means in terms of each distortion. I find it easier to just make either a level or decidedly slanted line and then, to indicate the severity of the particular distortion, simply write the word *slight, moderate,* or *marked* (or an abbreviation for one of these) at one end of the slanted line. If you want to use another system, such as "S," "M," or "L" to indicate small, medium, or large amounts of line slant, that's fine; use any system that makes sense to you, as long as you're consistent and can remember later on what your notes and abbreviations mean. Once you decide on your marking system, you can use that system to indicate the degree of severity on any of the other measurements you'll be taking from here on.

If your partner's arches are equal—both normal, both totally dropped, or both partially dropped (but equally so)—you're ready to proceed to the next step. If, however, your partner's arches are distinctly different—one normal and one dropped, or both dropped, but to different degrees—you need to pause here for a moment. If your partner happens to wear orthotics (arch support inserts worn in shoes), have your partner take those orthotics out of the shoes and stand on them for the rest of the evaluation of the front and back of the body. If no orthotics are available, have your partner put on a pair of shoes with built-in arch supports or inserts, such as good athletic shoes, and wear them while you are taking the front and back measurements. When we get to measurements from the side, your partner should remove the shoes or orthotics and stand in bare feet again.

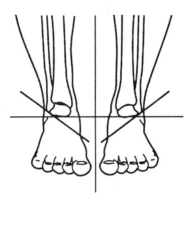

Figure 7-3a

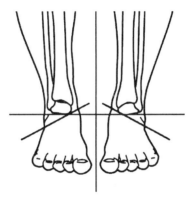

Figure 7-3b

Figure 7-3

The reason for this is simple: If one arch is dropped more than the other, that whole side of the body will drop with it, causing measurements of points higher on the body to appear more tilted than they otherwise would. By having your partner wear orthotics or shoes with equal arch supports, you create a situation where the arches are temporarily made equal, thereby taking the arch differential out of the equation when trying to determine the cause of any remaining tilts in the pelvis or shoulders.

Pelvis

Before measuring the pelvis, it is important to reposition the feet so that the heels are about 3 to 4 inches apart. A sheet of paper or piece of wood cut to a 4-inch length can be used as a guide by placing it on the floor and having your partner bring the inner edges of his or her heels and feet up against it on each side. In a case where your partner has a relatively small frame and a narrow pelvis, the distance between the feet can be decreased to about 3 inches. If you have no means of measuring and have to guess, it is better to have the heels a little too close than too far apart. Don't agonize over this distance, though; if you're off slightly on the distance, it won't make an appreciable difference in your measurement as long as the feet aren't more than about 4 inches apart. Once the feet are in position, make sure that your partner is standing with both knees straight, neither flexed (buckled forward) nor hyperextended (buckled slightly backward).

The first measurement you'll take at the pelvis is on either side of the iliac crest, the ridge along the top of the pelvis on either side. To measure the iliac crest, kneel in front of your partner and, with your hands positioned as shown in Figure 7-4a, place the tips of your fingers on top of the iliac crest on each side of the pelvis. Be sure to keep your fingers locked straight and parallel to the floor. Remember to kneel in front of your partner and keep your eyes at precisely the level of your measurement. See if one side appears higher than the other; if so, mark it accordingly on the chart, with a slanted line that indicates which side is higher (see Figure 7-4b). If the two sides appear even, just mark a level line across the top of the pelvis on the chart.

The second measurement at the pelvis is taken at the top of the greater trochanter, the knob of bone at the top of the femur or thigh bone. Depending on the height of your partner, drop your hands down roughly 3 to 5 inches from the top of the iliac crests, which you just measured. If you press in with the flat pads of the fingers, you can usually feel the trochanter as a bony lump. Once you locate the trochanters, point your fingers and press first straight in above them, then down on top of them, just as you did on the iliac crests (see Figure 7-5a). Mark the trochanters as either level or tilted, just as you did for the iliac crests (see Figure 7-5b).

If you have trouble locating the trochanters, try putting the flat pads of your fingers in position by pressing in gently on either side of the pelvis, about 3 to 5 inches from the top of the iliac crests, then either have your partner do a slight knee bend and stand up again, or else cause your partner to sway side to side by gently pushing the pelvis right and left with your hands (I've nicknamed this maneuver the "hula hips.") Using either method, you should be able to feel the bony lump of the trochanter moving under your fingers; once you've located the trochanters, you can place your fingers in position, pressing down on the top surface of the trochanters, and take your measurement.

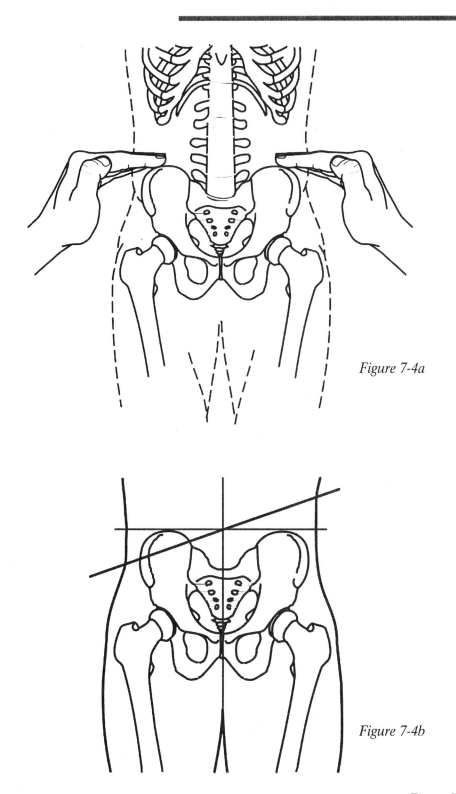

Figure 7-4a

Figure 7-4b

Figure 7-4

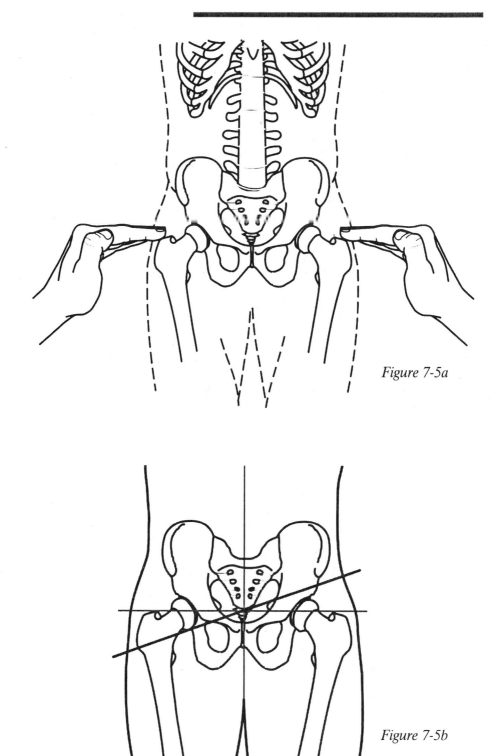

Figure 7-5a

Figure 7-5b

Figure 7-5

Shoulders

The shoulders are measured in very much the same way as the iliac crests, except that a different hand position is used. First, locate the lateral (outer) end of the clavicle or collarbone on each side. If you use flat hands to palpate it, it should feel like a bony lump on the top of each shoulder about 1 1/2 inches to 2 inches in from the end of each shoulder. An alternate way to locate those points is to place your fingertips on the upper surface of your partner's collarbones, then slide your fingers outward along each collarbone until you fall off the end onto the bone at the end of the shoulder. The bony prominence on either side that your finger just fell off is the end of the collarbone, the point you're looking for.

Now place the sides of your index fingers (pads of the fingers toward you) on the bony end of the shoulder so that the ends of your fingers are just behind the lateral ends of each collarbone (see Figure 7-6a). Do *not* try to make your fingers point directly at each other, as that will only tend to confuse you; just make sure that both fingers are perfectly horizontal. Be sure to adjust your posture so that your eyes are exactly at the height of your fingers, then check your measurement. If the two fingers appear to be at the same height, mark the shoulders as level; if they are at different heights, mark the chart accordingly with a slanted line (see Figure 7 6b).

Again, in order to avoid "creating" the measurement you think will be there, or if your first measurement is not obviously correct, try the technique of looking away, adjusting the position of your index fingers as needed until they feel as though they're in the same location on both sides, then quickly turn back and look at the measurement. As always, if need be, feel free to remeasure as often as necessary until you get a measurement that seems accurate.

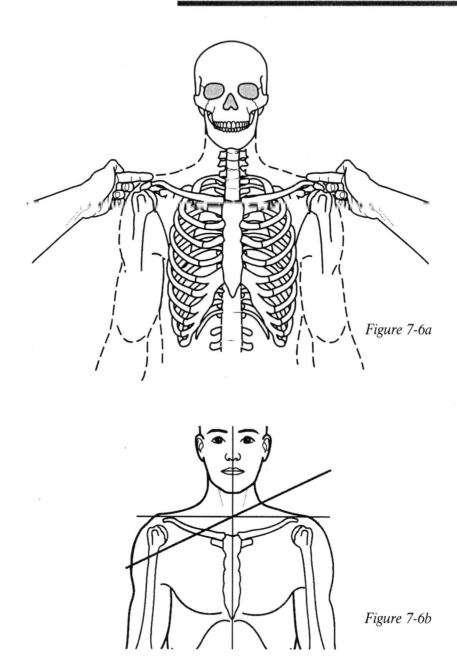

Figure 7-6a

Figure 7-6b

Figure 7-6

Rotation

At this point it is important to make sure that your partner's feet are parallel and positioned with the backs of the heels lined up against a straight edge, such as the edge of a magazine or a line in the floor, so that neither foot is in front of the other. As noted in our earlier discussion of rotational distortion, this ensures that your partner doesn't start out with a natural rotation; if, for example, the right foot is slightly forward of the left, the torso will of course rotate to the left.

Next, you need to find the point of bone, one on each side of the pelvis, known to anatomists as the anterior superior iliac spine, or ASIS for short. You can try to find this first on yourself by pressing in near the outside edges of the front of your pelvis with the pads of your fingers; you should feel that point of bone, the ASIS, under your fingers on each side of the pelvis. To locate your partner's right ASIS, with your partner standing sideways in front of you and facing to your right, put your left hand behind the right side of your partner's pelvis for support, then use the pads of the fingers of your right hand to gently feel for the bony point on the outer edge of the front of the pelvis. Next, find the left ASIS in the same manner. Once you've located them both, gently place the pads of your thumbs right on the very front of the two bony points, keeping your thumbs straight and pointing straight across the body.

Now, standing in front of your partner, get your eyes as far forward and over your thumbs as you reasonably can, then look down at your thumbs (see Figure 7-7a). The solid lines show the hands and thumbs in position on the pelvis; the dotted lines are there just to indicate where the shoulders and head would be, if viewed from above. See if one thumb is slightly closer to you, the other slightly farther away. If so, because the heels should still be equidistant from you, being on a straight line, the pelvis is rotated. If one side of the pelvis is forward, draw and fill in a small triangle on the same side of the pelvis on the chart as a kind of arrowhead to remind you that this side is swinging forward and around toward the other side (see Figure 7-7b); if neither side is forward, you can either mark nothing or make a light "X" on each side of the pelvis, just as we discussed when we measured the arches, as a reminder to yourself that you checked them and they were "x-actly" where they were supposed to be

The next step is to do the same thing at the shoulders. Gently position your thumbs on the front of the shoulders so that they rest on the upper part of the upper arm bone or humerus on either side (see Figure 7-8a). Now, just as you did at the pelvis, try to see if one shoulder is forward in relationship to the other. Sometimes you can easily see this by just looking straight at your thumbs from the front and using your depth perception. If you can't tell clearly by looking from the front, then you'll need to try to look down somewhat from

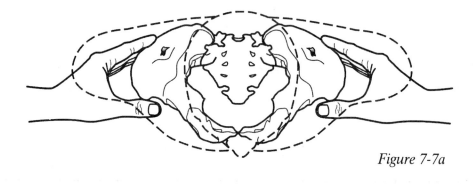

Figure 7-7a

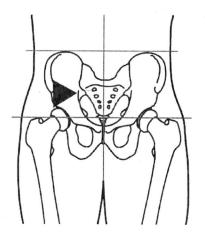

Figure 7-7b

Figure 7-7

above, much as you did when looking for rotation in the pelvis. If you are significantly taller than your partner, this is easy enough to do just by moving in closer and looking down at your thumbs from above. However, if you aren't enough taller than your partner to be able to do this, you'll need to stand on a stool or small ladder to allow you to have that view from above. Once you determine the relative position of the shoulders, you can mark the shoulders in exactly the same way you marked the pelvis, with either a filled-in triangle on the more forward shoulder, pointing to the other side (see Figure 7-8b) or a light "X" on each shoulder to indicate that they were checked and were "x-actly" equal.

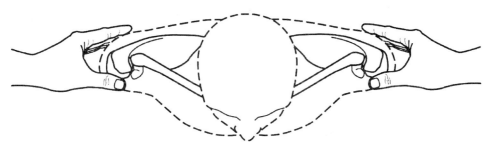

Figure 7-8a

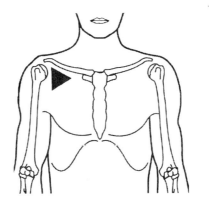

Figure 7-8b

Figure 7-8

Arms and Hands

Leaving the feet in this heels-even position, it's time now to check your partner's arms and hands. Step back and take a general look at your partner's arm and hand position. In proper posture, the hands should hang at the sides of the body with the backs of the hands facing exactly to your partner's right and left, and so that when you stand in front of your partner you can see through the gap between the thumb and fingers on each side (see Figure 2-1). If this is what you see, that's great; just put a light "X" on each hand to remind yourself that you've checked it and you're done. Not uncommonly, however, the hands are found partially around toward the front of the thighs, and with the backs of the hands facing more toward the front than to the sides (see Figure 7-9a). This comes from the shoulders being pulled forward, usually from working for extended periods with the hands in front of the body as so many of us do in our society (typing on computers, driving, writing at a desk, playing piano, etc.).

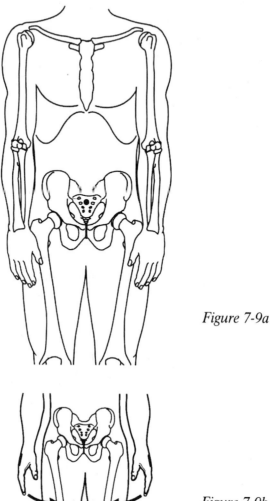

Figure 7-9a

Figure 7-9b

Figure 7-9

Sometimes you may find that, although the hands are not around toward the front of the thighs but are in fact at the sides of the thighs where they are supposed to be, they are nonetheless somewhat turned so that the palms of the hands are facing slightly, or even totally, backward (see Figure 7-10a). This can be caused by rotation of the arm at one of two points. If it occurs at the shoulder, it's called medial or internal rotation of the humerus or upper arm; if the upper arm position is normal and the rotation occurs only below the elbow, it's called pronation of the forearms (as discussed in Chapter 5).

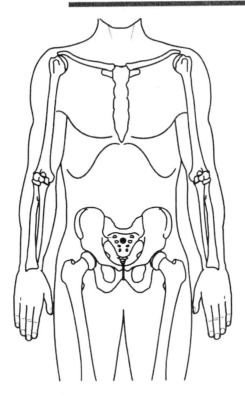

Figure 7-10a

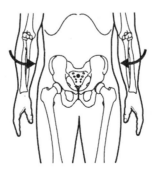

Figure 7-10b

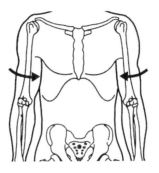

Figure 7-10c

Figure 7-10

Many times the forward shoulders, medial rotation of the upper arm, and pronated forearms are found together in various combinations, especially, for example, in people who work at computers for extended periods of time. In order to get a sense of which distortion(s) are present, have your partner gently pull the shoulders back until the elbows come around to the sides of the body, roughly above where the stripe would be on a pair of uniform pants. If the hands are now in proper position, with the backs of the hands facing directly out to each side, the problem is that the shoulders have been drawn forward. To record this on your partner's chart, place an arrow under the affected hand(s) on the chart (see Figure 7-9b).

If, however, the hands are still turned with the backs of the hands somewhat forward, either the upper arms are medially rotated or the forearms are pronated. To distinguish between the two, look at the elbows. If the creases of the elbows face almost forward, the upper arms are probably in pretty good alignment and the hands are turned due to pronation, which occurs below the elbow. You can mark this on your partner's chart by placing a curved arrow across the forearm of the affected hand(s) to show the inward rotation (see Figure 7-10b). However, if the elbow creases face more in toward the sides of the body and the elbows point more outward on each side than backward, medial rotation of the upper arms is the likely culprit. To confirm this, have your partner rotate the upper arms so that the elbow creases face almost forward; if this solves the problem by making the backs of the hands now face out to the sides, you've confirmed that the distortion was caused by the medial rotation of the upper arms. You can note this by placing a curved arrow across the upper arm of the affected hand(s) to show the inward rotation (see Figure 7-10c). If correcting the medial rotation helps but the backs of the hands are still facing somewhat forward, the forearms are also pronated.

Although they're not as common as pronation and medial rotation of the upper arm, the opposite conditions, supination of the forearm and lateral rotation of the upper arm, can also occur. In supination, instead of the normal hand position at the sides, the hands appear turned so that the palms are facing somewhat forward, rather than backward, as in pronation. If this is the case, and if the elbow creases appear to be in their normal position, mark the chart accordingly (see Figure 7-11a). This slight palm-forward position of the hand can also be caused by lateral rotation of the upper arm, so if the shoulders appear to be drawn back and the elbow crease appears to face either more directly forward than normal or even slightly outward, the upper arm is laterally rotated. In this case, mark the chart accordingly (see Figure 7-11b).

Finally, let's look at the hands themselves. If the fingers of the hands are noticeably curved or curled inward, instead of being relatively straight as they

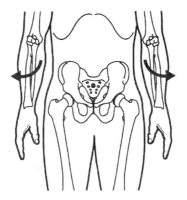

Figure 7-11a

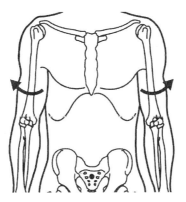

Figure 7-11b

Figure 7-11

hang by the sides, the finger flexors are tight. This is frequently caused by keeping the fingers in a flexed position for an extended period of time, as in typing or playing the piano, and also by extended periods of tight gripping, as in working with tools. If the fingers are flexed, mark the chart accordingly (see Figure 7-12).

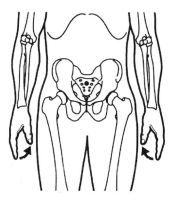

Figure 7-12

Please remember, though, as stated earlier in the chapter, that these conditions can occur in a variety of combinations that only a skilled examiner can sort out, so don't feel as though you have to become expert at these nuances to succeed. If you do your best and trust your measurements, you'll be surprised how accurate a picture of the body you'll be able to create. And remember that you're only looking for obvious postural distortions. If you check two or three times and can't tell if something is distorted, it's probably not significant for our purposes in this book. Just mark it with a light "X" to show you've checked it, move on the next point, and enjoy unraveling the mysteries of the human body.

Chapter 8

A Keen Eye, Part 2:
Measuring From the Back

When Mike came for his first appointment, he was nearly at his wit's end. At age 34, after years of fruitless search for relief of his low back pain, he'd finally gone to one of the best-known back clinics in the country. After doing a complete evaluation, the back specialists gave him three choices: "We can fuse your lumbar spine, we can cauterize the nerve so you won't feel the pain, or we can do a spinal tap on you every 90 days." He thought they were crazy, walked out, and shortly thereafter came to me for evaluation.

After doing a postural analysis, I explained to Mike that his left femur was about 1/4-inch shorter than his right, causing his pelvis to tilt to the left and forcing his back muscles to be in constant contraction in order to pull his torso to the right and hold him upright. I worked briefly on his tight back muscles, offered him a piece of 1/4-inch thick material to test inside his shoe, which he was more than ready to do, and sent him home. When he came back the following week, he was feeling much better, so I continued releasing the muscles that had been so tight and painful for so many years. Because his schedule was so busy, he said he'd call me shortly, as soon as things quieted down, to set up his third appointment. Nine months later, I was talking to Lou, the friend who'd referred Mike, and asked, "What ever happened to Mike?" "Oh, he's doing great," Lou said. "Well, that's nice to hear, but he still needs more work," I countered, to which Lou replied, "Yeah, he knows that, and he is planning to come in, but he's feeling so good that he's just going to call you when he gets the time." After five years, I still haven't received that call.

Now that you've worked your way up the front of the body, taking measurements from the feet to the shoulders, it's both convenient and logical now to work your way down the back. Beginning at the shoulders, you'll use the same procedure you used when you measured the shoulders from the front, and at the same point. This may seem redundant, measuring the same points again, as you will at the pelvis also, but believe me, it's very worthwhile. Usually these second measurements just confirm what you found when you measured from the front, and that alone is helpful, as it gives you greater confidence in the accuracy of your measurements. Sometimes, however, taking these measurements from a different perspective can help you to refine or correct your previous measurements. This is particularly true of the shoulder measurement, as it is often easier to see the shoulder measurement clearly from the back than from the front.

Shoulders

Have your partner positioned just as you did when measuring from the front, with the feet no more than about 3 to 4 inches apart and both knees straight, neither flexed nor hyperextended. Then, as you did from the front, locate the lateral (outer) end of the clavicle or collarbone and place the sides of your index fingers, with the pads of the fingers toward you, on the bony end of the shoulder, just posterior to (behind) the lateral ends of each collarbone (see Figure 8-1a). Chart your findings accordingly on the shoulder line on the back view of the body, just as you did when measuring from the front.

Remember that to avoid creating a distortion, you shouldn't try to make your fingers point directly at each other, but instead just keep each finger perfectly horizontal on its own shoulder. Now position your body so that your eyes are exactly at the level of your fingers, then take your measurement and mark the chart just as you did when you measured from the front As always, it's good to use the technique of looking away, shifting your index fingers around as necessary until they feel as though they're in the same place on both sides, then quickly looking back at your fingers and taking the measurement.

When measuring from the back, it's always good to take a confirming measurement at the bottom point of the shoulder blade, known as the inferior angle of the scapula, as it is usually easy to feel and generally offers a clear and unambiguous reading. With your fingers positioned around the sides of the chest, point your thumbs toward the spine and let them rest against the back just below the inferior angle on each side. Now, keeping the thumbs perfectly horizontal, slide them up the back until their upper edges just touch the inferior angle on each side (see Figure 8-1b). As always, remember not to try to make your thumbs point at each other, but instead keep them horizontal on each side. Now get your eyes down to the level of your thumbs and note whether the inferior angles are level, or if one is higher, and mark your chart accordingly (see Figure 8-1c).

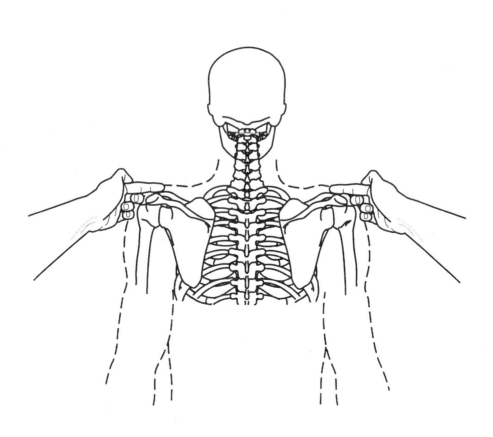

Figure 8-1a

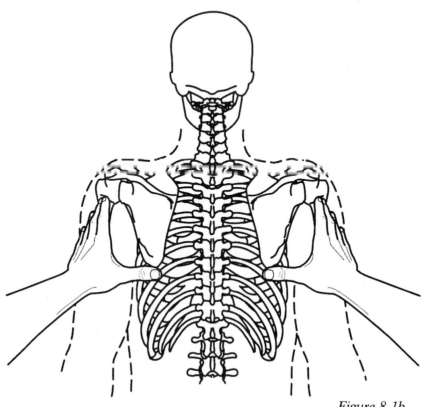

Figure 8-1b

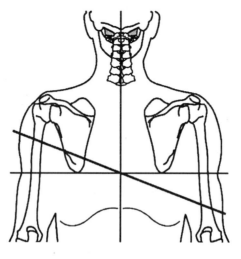

Figure 8-1c

Figure 8-1

Except in rare circumstances, the inferior angle measurement should match the shoulder measurement, meaning that whether the shoulders are level or tilted, the inferior angle should also be level or tilted in the same direction. If the two measurements don't agree, try taking both measurements again; in all probability, this will resolve the discrepancy. Although it is in fact possible that a difference in the two measurements could be correct, that can be true only when either the two scapulae or shoulder blades are in fact physically different in size or when one of the two scapulae is markedly rotated out of position. In my experience, though, the first of these conditions is quite rare and the second one is both uncommon and usually easy to notice, so it's always advisable to recheck these two measurements if they disagree.

Pelvis

The measurement at the iliac crest is the same as from the front. Again, kneel behind your partner and, with your fingers locked straight and parallel to the floor, position the tips of your fingers on top of the iliac crest on each side of the pelvis (see Figure 8-2). Position your eyes right at the level of your measurement, then see if one side appears higher than the other, or if they appear level. Chart your findings accordingly on the iliac crest line on the back view of the pelvis, just as you did when measuring from the front.

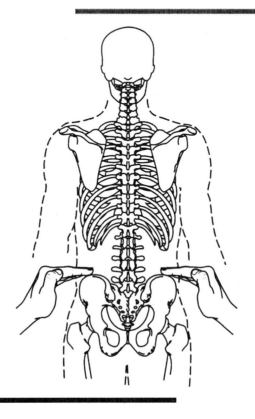

Figure 8-2

Now remeasure at the top of the greater trochanter, the upper end of the femur or thigh bone. Move your hands down about 3 to 5 inches (depending on the height of your partner) from the iliac crests. Just as you did when measuring from the front, first press in with the flat part of the fingers to locate the trochanters on either side of the pelvis. Once you've found them, point your fingers and press in above the trochanters, then down on top of them (see Figure 8-3). Chart your findings accordingly on the trochanter line on the back view of the pelvis, just as you did when measuring from the front. As before, if you have trouble locating the trochanters, try having your partner do either the slight knee bend or the "hula hips" sway to help you locate the trochanters.

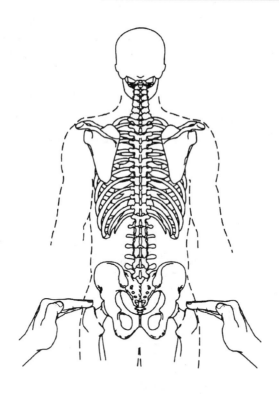

Figure 8-3

Ankles

For this measurement you want your partner standing in a relaxed, "normal" position in bare feet, so if you found an apparent difference in the arches and had your partner stand on orthotics or put on shoes, the orthotics or shoes need to be removed at this point. Now look at the Achilles tendon, the band that runs up from the calcaneus or heel bone to the back of the leg. Ideally, it should appear to be essentially straight (as shown in Figure 8-4a). If, however, the Achilles tendon is bowed inward (see Figure 8-4b) on either side, it indicates that the arch on that foot has flattened out, at least to some degree. Although you have already measured the arches directly from the front, this measurement provides a helpful confirmation of your reading at the arches. Chart your findings accordingly on the ankle line on the back view of the body, just as you did when measuring from the front.

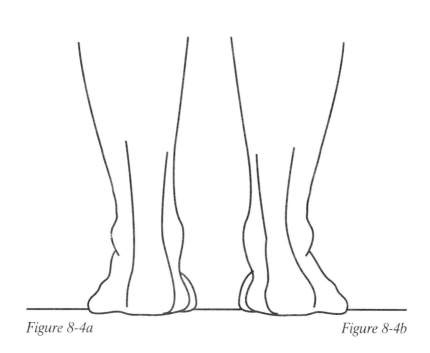

Figure 8-4a   *Figure 8-4b*

Figure 8-4

There's one other measurement at the ankles that doesn't fall under measuring from the front, back, or side, so this is as good a point as any to take care of it. Have your partner lie supine (face up) and barefoot on the floor, then look at the soles (plantar surfaces) of your partner's feet. Ideally they should be essentially vertical, at a right angle to the floor, but it is common to find the ankles plantar flexed, meaning that they are tilted so that the feet point somewhat away from the head. This is a common source of calf pain, particularly among dancers, figure skaters, or sprinters who spend a lot of time on their toes, which causes the muscles in the back of the lower leg to actively contract, and among people who regularly wear, or have worn, high heel shoes or boots, thus keeping the posterior calf muscles in a passively shortened position to which those muscles gradually adapt. If the soles of the feet are roughly at right angles to the floor, simply mark an "X" just to the outside of each of the feet of the postural chart figure (Figure 2-1) marked "Front" to show that you've checked them and that they're "x-actly" correct. However, if the sole of either foot is tilted away from the head, mark the chart with a "PF" (see Figure 8-5) to indicate that the ankle is plantar flexed.

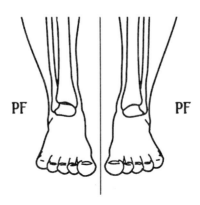

Figure 8-5

Chapter 9

A Keen Eye, Part 3:
Measuring From the Side

When Denny came in for his first appointment, his major complaint was a persistent, nagging pain in his lower left abdomen, the cause of which had so far eluded his doctors. Because he was in some significant discomfort when he arrived, I hurried our intake interview slightly in order to be able to work on him sooner, and I forgot to notice what he had put down under "Occupation." As I measured him from the side during the postural evaluation, I found that his pelvis was strongly rotated forward on both sides. Later, when I checked the psoas major muscles in his abdomen, the right one was very tender, but the left was excruciating.

It was then that I remembered to ask him what he did for a living. When he told me that he was a professional pool player, everything became clear. All that time spent bent over at the waist, particularly over his left leg, had caused his hip flexor muscles to adaptively shorten and tighten, as a result of which trigger points in his left psoas major muscle were firing into his abdomen and causing his pain. I explained to Denny that he didn't have to quit his chosen profession, but that if he wanted to stay out of pain he'd have to stretch his hip flexor muscles and strengthen his hip extensor muscles every day to counterbalance the constant hip flexion his job demanded. Once he started his home therapy program, his abdominal pain gradually disappeared and has not returned.

In order to measure from the side, have your partner turn sideways to you, making sure that your partner's feet are roughly 3 to 4 inches apart with the heels lined up, so that neither heel is further back than the other. If you don't line up the heels, the body will naturally turn toward the heel that's farther back, distorting one of your measurements. Make sure that your partner stays facing straight forward while you're measuring, again to prevent distortion. Finally, if you had your partner wearing orthotics or shoes to correct for uneven arches, your partner should have removed them when you checked the arches from the back by looking at the Achilles tendon; be sure that your partner keeps them off and stands in bare feet for the side measurements.

Shoulder/Head Alignment

For the sake of discussion, let's assume you're measuring your partner's right side first. Look at your partner from the side and see if the right shoulder and ear appear to be in line, one directly above the other. If your partner's hair is covering the ear, try to move the hair out of the way or, if possible, have your partner tie it back or pull it up so that you can see the ear clearly.

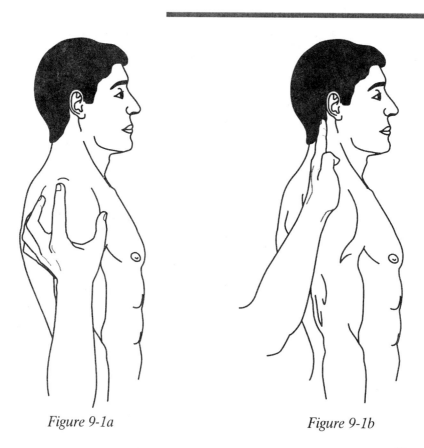

Figure 9-1a   Figure 9-1b

Figure 9-1

First, close your right thumb and fingers gently on the end of the shoulder and locate the bone that sits across the very end of the shoulder above the arm. Lightly hold that bone between your thumb and middle finger to measure the full width of the bone, then touch your index finger to the shoulder midway between your thumb and middle finger (see Figure 9-1a). This is a rough way of determining the middle of the shoulder so that you can start from the same point on both sides.

Now turn your hand and rest its pinkie edge on this shoulder midpoint with the fingertips pointing toward the head (see Figure 9-1b). Making sure to get your eye directly in line with your hand, look straight along your hand, and see where that line would contact the head. To verify this, move your hand straight forward and see where your fingertips meet your partner's head. Ideally, your hand should point toward, or run into, the external auditory meatus or "ear hole." Quite often, though, the line from the shoulder will actually be behind or in front of the ear hole (see Figure 9-1b). You can either estimate how far in front or in back of the ear hole your finger is, or hold up a ruler with your other hand and measure the distance from the ear hole to your finger, then mark it on the chart. Remember that, because your line of sight from the shoulder indicates roughly the point where the ear hole should be, you want to mark the chart to indicate which way the head has moved from that point (see Figure 9-2). Now walk around your partner and repeat the measurement on the left side. I should add that, because this measurement technique involves moving the hand toward the head, that movement increases the possibility for error, so I always double or triple measure on each side to assure myself of a reliable measurement.

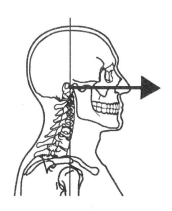

Figure 9-2

Pelvis

Measurement of the pelvis from the side is used to determine whether the pelvis has rotated anteriorly or posteriorly. This is very important information to know in getting yourself out of pain, but it is the hardest technique to explain in a book intended for the general public. When measuring someone in my office, I check several bony landmarks and I use a device called a goniometer, a kind of glorified protractor with arms, to measure the angle of pelvic inclination, as it's called, but most readers are not likely to have a goniometer handy or know how to use it. Still, there are ways to get a rough idea of the pelvic angle, and that will suffice for our purposes here.

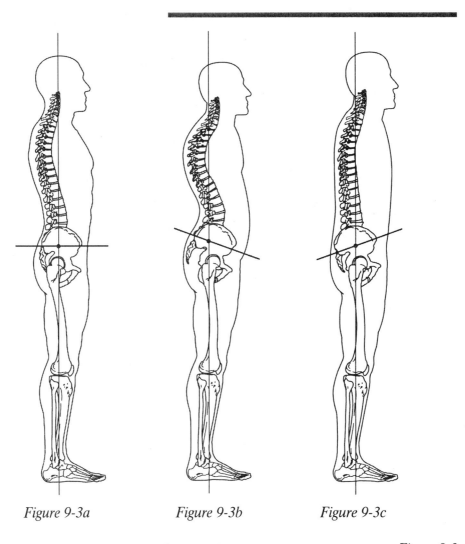

Figure 9-3a   Figure 9-3b   Figure 9-3c

Figure 9-3

In Figure 9-3 you see illustrations of normal pelvic alignment, anterior rotation, and posterior rotation. Remember that the normal pelvic angle ranges from level to very slightly anterior, and it differs in men and women (see Figure 3-2), with the normal range of tilt in women (5 degrees to 10 degrees) being slightly more anterior than in men (0 degrees to 5 degrees). Also, please note that these "normal" angles apply only to adults; it is natural for children to have that somewhat anteriorly-tilted, "pot-bellied" look when they are young. About age 10 to 12, however, the body begins to take on its adult alignment, so that even in a teenager the pelvic angle should ideally fall in the ranges shown.

Notice how in the illustration of anterior rotation the pelvis has tipped forward, causing the low back to have to curve markedly in order to keep the torso upright. That exaggerated lumbar curve, known as a lordosis, is usually a telltale sign of an anteriorly rotated pelvis. Notice also whether your partner's waistline appears to be tilted down in front, and likewise with the belt or the top of the pants, another possible indicator of anterior pelvic rotation. Please remember, though, that although the angle of clothing is a possible confirmation it is not always reliable and should never be used as the only indicator when making your judgment, because clothing can shift or be worn askew. Still, it is worth noting in conjunction with the lumbar curve. Also, when the pelvis is in anterior rotation the abdominal muscles tend to be stretched and weak, resulting in a protruding abdomen.

By contrast, the illustration of posterior rotation shows the pelvis tipped backward, causing the low back to flatten out, and that flatness usually extends up toward the middle of the spine, sometimes even reaching as high as the area between the shoulder blades. The waistline of the body—and frequently (but not necessarily) the waistband or belt line of the clothing—may be tilted slightly down in back.

To measure your partner's pelvic rotation, first make sure that you can get a clear and unobstructed view of the midsection of the body, from the bottom of the shoulder blades and lower chest to the top of the pelvis. If your partner is wearing a shirt or top that obstructs your view of this area, have your partner either remove the shirt, if consistent with modesty, or else tuck up or pin up the bottom edge of the shirt so that you have a clear view of the abdomen and the lower half of the back. Now, with your partner standing sideways to you, note whether the pelvis appears to be tilted forward or back. Be sure to check both the degree of curvature of the lower back (the area just above the pelvis) and the apparent tilt of the waistband or belt. If it's not clear at first, refer to the illustrations in Figure 9-3 to get a clearer picture of what you're looking for.

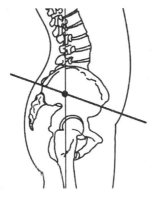

Figure 9-4a

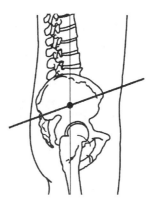

Figure 9-4b

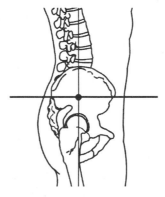

Figure 9-4c

Figure 9-4

Remember what we said earlier: Don't agonize over fine distinctions! If the pelvis clearly appears to be rotated either anteriorly or posteriorly—in other words, more or less than the ranges of tilt shown in Figure 3-2—mark it as such (see Figure 9-4a and Figure 9-4b). Remember also that these ranges mean that, for a woman, even a level pelvis is actually slightly posteriorly rotated, because a female pelvis is supposed to be very slightly tilted, at least 5 degrees forward. If you can't tell—if, for example, the low back appears to have just a normal, slight curve, rather than a more pronounced one, and the waistband or belt appears to be either level or only very slightly down in front—just mark it as normal with a level line (see Figure 9-4c) or an "X" to show that it was "x-actly" where it should be. When it comes to planning your work for this area, we'll usually treat an unsure "normal" reading as a possible slight anterior reading, unless we have other information to the contrary.

Congratulations! That does it; you now have all the information you need to plan your pain-relief program. Although there are lots of other points that could be measured and notes that could be made, the measurements you've just taken will give you all the basic information you need to effectively treat your pain. Now that you have your chart covered with all these strange marks and lines, let's figure out what it all means.

Section III

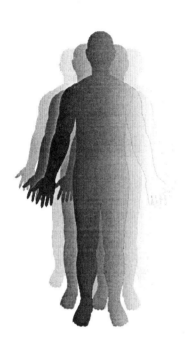

Getting Rid of
Your Pain

Chapter 10

Before You Begin:
Mastering the Principles of Postural Pain Relief

Carl and Stacy met at a cycling event and both loved to work out, so it was hardly surprising that after they got married they went to the gym together all the time. Stacy had come to see me first, referred by her personal trainer, who was concerned because she had gradually started to experience back pain and wanted me to check her for any postural distortions. After completing her postural evaluation, I asked Stacy to give me a copy of her workout routine. It was a nicely balanced workout, which would have been fine except that Stacy didn't have a nicely balanced body. Her pelvis was rotated sharply forward to about 18 degrees on both sides, tightening her hip flexors and low back muscles, yet she was doing several exercises that specifically strengthened those very muscles that were already too tight! In order to restore her body to postural balance, we changed her workout routine to stretch her tight muscles and only strengthen her over-stretched muscles. At our next session, she was delighted with how the new workout routine made her back feel, so she promptly made an appointment for Carl, who for the last several years had been having bouts of pain in his upper back, shoulder, neck, and head. He, too, was doing some of the wrong exercises, in his case exercises that would strengthen his already-too-tight chest muscles that were pulling his shoulders forward, thus causing his pain syndrome. Once we revised Carl's workout to only stretch his chest muscles, while strengthening his upper and middle back muscles, he, too, was able to steadily diminish, and finally eliminate, his pain.

Reading your postural chart and planning your pain relief program is a lot easier than it may seem at first, and once you understand the basic concepts involved you'll see that it's really just a matter of using logic and common sense. Simply put, what we're trying to determine is which muscles are out of balance, either too tight and in need of stretching or too loose and in need of strengthening. By looking at the distortions you've marked on your chart and understanding what they imply about your muscles, you can intelligently create a personalized stretching and exercise program to relieve your musculoskeletal pain.

If you're wondering whether you'll have to go back to school and get a "degree in muscles" in order to understand your chart, fear not. When I present this material to healthcare professionals, it's only natural to use lots of anatomical terms and to analyze the distortions muscle by muscle, but that simply won't work here. As a result, once you grasp the underlying principles of chart-reading laid out in the following pages, you'll be given a simple, visual system for constructing your own program step by step. (If you're interested in learning this work in greater detail, whether for professional or personal use, please see the Appendix for information about training seminars.)

Remember the Laws

Whenever you study a postural chart, be sure to keep in mind the basic laws and principles we discussed earlier. If you understand those laws, it will help you to understand why your postural distortions have occurred and how to go about correcting them. Here's a quick refresher of the main points we covered in Chapter 1:

▸ Muscles only contract and pull; they can't push.

▸ Joints function because muscles work in pairs of opposing muscles or muscle groups. When muscles on one side of a joint become weaker or stronger than those on the other side, the stronger muscles pull the joint out of alignment, creating postural distortion.

▸ When the ends of a muscle get closer together, the muscle adaptively shortens and strengthens; when the ends of a muscle get farther apart, the muscle develops stretch weakening.

▸ Gravity pulls body parts toward the earth, causing opposing muscles to contract in order to compensate and attempt to restore postural balance.

▸ Your center of gravity is the center of your body's mass—your "balance point"—and your body instinctively contracts muscles to keep that "balance point" over your base of support (that is, between your feet and between the balls of your feet and the center of your heels) in order to keep you from falling over.

▶ The Righting Reflex is that complex of instinctive reactions of the body that constantly adjusts your posture to keep your eyes level with the horizon, your face forward, and your center of gravity over your base of support.

Rules for Using Your Chart

Keeping in mind those laws, you're now ready to take a look at your chart. Here are some simplified rules for using your chart to create your own pain relief stretching and exercise program:

▶ If horizontal lines are tilted, your workout needs to make them level.

▶ If the pelvis is rotated forward or backward out of the normal range, your workout needs to rotate it in the opposite direction until it reaches, and remains in, the normal range.

▶ If the pelvis, shoulders, and/or head are rotated to one side, your workout needs to rotate each of them in the opposite direction until they all are even and face straight ahead.

▶ If the arms or legs are internally or externally rotated, your workout needs to rotate them in the opposite direction until they reach, and remain in, a neutral position.

▶ If a part of the body is out of position, thereby creating postural distortion, the muscles in the direction it moved **toward** are **too tight; stretch** them. The muscles in the direction it moved **away from** are **too weak; strengthen** them.

Look at Your Life

At this point it's important to take a moment to examine both your life history and your daily activities. After all, these are the sources that have created, and every day are continuing to create, your postural distortions. As an example, let's look at Ruby's case. Ten years before she came to see me, Ruby's car was struck in the driver's side door by another car, causing the door to buckle inward and hit her in the left side of her chest, abdomen, and pelvis, as well as causing a side-to-side whiplash injury in her neck. Although the doctors at the hospital found no major injuries and released her, not only did the whiplash result in serious muscle pain in her neck, shoulders, and head, but the trauma to her left side caused the muscles on that side to tighten, thus lowering her left shoulder. That low shoulder went unnoticed and untreated, and it was still lower 10 years later when Ruby walked into my office. In this case, Ruby's distortion had been caused primarily by a past physical trauma.

Remember the example in Chapter 1 of Mark, the businessman who drove all day with his right elbow leaning on the center console of his car and his left hand on the top of the steering wheel? By spending so much time with his shoulders tilted, his rib cage crunched down on the right, and his head pulled back up toward the left, Mark had tightened his muscles and created his postural distortion just in the course of his daily activities.

These are just two examples of the kinds of major events or mundane, everyday activities that can lead to postural distortion, and it's important to discover, if you can, the original cause or causes of the distortions you just found in your measurements. If a distortion was caused by a one-time, major event, as in the case of Ruby's car accident, it is reasonable to expect that, once you correct the distortions caused by that event, the correction is likely to stay unless you should happen to suffer another similar major injury. If, however, the distortion was caused by some common activity in your everyday life—for example, the way you drive, the way you sit at your desk, the kind of work you do, the way you sleep, even the exercises you do at the gym—any correction is not likely to last long, because you'll be recreating the distortion every day when you engage in those activities. Consequently, it's important to try to understand the root cause of any postural distortion, because only by eliminating that root cause will the postural distortion stay corrected and your musculoskeletal pain be kept from coming back.

In my experience, although the untreated effects of past injuries certainly can and do cause postural distortion and pain, by far the most common source of postural distortion and chronic pain is the way we sit, stand, sleep, and move in the course of our ordinary, everyday lives. Consequently, it's important to try to think about all the various postures you habitually assume, many of them more or less unconscious, during both your waking and sleeping hours to see if you can find any that are contributing to your distortion and your pain. Do the best you can with this "life examination" for now, correcting any postural bad habits you can find, and we'll visit this subject again later, after you've created your pain relief program.

Principles of Postural Pain Relief

Now that you've reviewed the laws of the body, learned the simplified rules for reading your chart, and examined your life for sources of your distortion and pain, it's time to create your personal pain relief program. Here, too, certain core principles exist and must be understood and followed if you want to be successful.

▶ **Remember the goal: To train your muscles to support you naturally in good posture without conscious effort.**

You can't be thinking of holding yourself in good posture at every moment of your life; after all, you have other things to do, a life to live, and you need to be able to focus your attention on those activities. Consequently, it's important to balance your musculature so that it naturally holds you in good posture, even when you're not thinking about it.

▶ **Until you achieve postural balance and pain relief, only stretch tight muscles and only strengthen weak muscles.**

If you stretch muscles that are already too stretched, it will increase your postural distortion and pain. Similarly, if you strengthen muscles that are already too tight, you can create new or increased pain.

▶ **Balanced workouts only work for posturally balanced bodies.**

If you strengthen unbalanced muscle groups equally, both muscle groups get stronger, but the imbalance of strength between them remains the same and the postural distortion doesn't change; the strengthened muscles now only further lock you into that distortion. It is disheartening to watch people working out in a gym and doing a "balanced" workout in which half the exercises are only making their postural distortions and pain problems worse. Your workout can become balanced when your posture becomes balanced, but not until then.

▶ **If you habitually shorten or tighten certain muscles each day in the course of your work or other daily activities, you have no choice but to regularly stretch them and tighten their opposing muscles if you want to avoid postural distortion and musculoskeletal pain.**

Simply put, because we naturally tighten or adaptively shorten some muscles more than others in the course of our daily activities, such muscularly unbalanced daily activities require workouts unbalanced in the opposite direction to regain and maintain good posture and to reduce or prevent pain. This particularly helps to prevent injuries in athletes, both professional and amateur, because a posturally balanced body is stronger and more resistant to being injured by the stresses placed on it by athletic competition.

▶ **If a postural distortion involves differences between the right and left sides of the body, it is usually necessary to strengthen a particular muscle or muscles on one side of the body while stretching the corresponding muscle(s) on the other side.**

In other words, if a muscle is tight on one side of the body but weak on the other side, thus creating a postural distortion, it is necessary to stretch only the tight side and strengthen only the weak side until you achieve postural balance and pain relief. Here, too, your workout can become balanced when your posture becomes balanced, but not until then.

▶ **To simply halt the gradual increase in postural distortion and pain as a result of daily activities, it is necessary to exert an equal amount of energy in the direction opposite that of the distortion; to actually reverse and eliminate the existing distortion requires an even greater (unequal) input of energy in that opposite direction.**

For instance, if you spend all day working at a desk or computer and your shoulders have been pulled forward because your chest muscles have adaptively shortened, you will need to put at least enough work into stretching your chest muscles and strengthening your weakened upper back muscles to counterbalance the daily "desk workout" that's tightening your chest muscles each day and thereby keep your distortion and pain from getting worse. If, however, you want to do more than that, if you want to actually reverse the distortion and bring your shoulders back into their correct postural position, you'll need to put still more effort into your corrective stretches and exercise (that is, more repetitions or sets, added weight or resistance, greater workout frequency, and so on). Although the exact point at which you precisely balance your daily activities is impossible to calculate exactly, you can begin with a workout strongly unbalanced in the direction of correcting your existing distortion. Then, once your shoulders are back in proper alignment, you can change to a less unbalanced workout that will keep your chest and back muscles balanced and your shoulders correctly positioned.

▶ **If, despite what was said above, you just can't bear to strengthen only the loose muscles or stretch only the tight muscles, always do at least four times as many of the "correct" exercises or stretches than the "incorrect" ones until you achieve postural balance and pain relief.**

Continuing with our example of the tight chest muscles, the fastest way to correct this distortion and relieve your pain is to stretch only the chest muscles and strengthen only the upper back muscles. Every now and then I have a client who says something along the lines of, "It just feels weird to only do stretching on one side of the body and only strengthening on the other. Can't I do at least some of each on both sides?" Although my usual response to them is a gentle, "If you want to get out of pain, what part of 'No' don't you understand?", I know that some people just have a tough time with this idea. In such cases, in the example of the chest muscles, I tell them that for every time they strengthen their already tight chest muscles, they have to strengthen their weak upper back muscles at least four times as much, and for every time they stretch their already weak upper back muscles they have to stretch their tight chest muscles at least four times as much. Although this ratio can change once the shoulders have moved back into position, it's important to create a strong imbalance in the workout program in the direction of correcting the postural distortion. Always remember, though, that it's far better and faster to stretch only the tight muscles and strengthen only the weak muscles until you achieve postural balance and pain relief.

▶ **Use this system of postural analysis to monitor your progress regularly and adjust your pain relief program as necessary.**

In the case of the forward shoulders, once your shoulders have moved back into correct postural alignment at your sides, you can start working in a little strengthening of the chest muscles and stretching of the back muscles, perhaps using a 3-to-1 ratio in favor of the original correction, then gradually progressing to perhaps 2 1/2-to-1, then 2-to-1, and so on. These ratios can be in terms of amount of resistance used, number of repetitions or sets, or any other measure of work done. If, as you gradually progress over time toward a more balanced workout, you begin to notice that your shoulders are starting to move forward again, that means that your workout has become too balanced and isn't correcting enough to counteract the daily tightening of your chest muscles. Simply start increasing your workout ratio to perhaps 3-to-1 or 4-to-1 until your shoulders return to their proper position. Better yet, to get them back in position quickly, stop all counter-corrective stretching and strengthening and follow the "stretch only the tight muscles, strengthen only the weak muscles" rule previously given.

Once your shoulders are again back in their correct position, you can start to rebalance the workout again, this time progressing more slowly and trying to notice where the balance point seems to be, the ratio at which your unbalanced corrective workout seems to balance out your unbalanced daily "desk workout" and keep your shoulders in position. Keep in mind, though, that if the nature and duration of your daily activities should change, your workout will need to change accordingly. The advantage of this system is that it's no trouble at all to monitor your posture and fine-tune your workout as needed.

▶ **Give your program time to work.**

Remember: It's probably taken you years of poor postural habits and miscellaneous injuries to create your present postural distortions and the resulting pain, so don't expect it all to vanish overnight. Although the many factors involved make it impossible to give any exact estimates of how long any particular condition will take to correct, it can be said with certainty that the more faithful and diligent you are in setting up and following your pain relief program, the faster you will see results. In general, distortions and muscular pain problems that are minor or of recent onset often resolve quickly, whereas major pain problems or those that have existed for many years typically take somewhat longer. Nevertheless, if you've already seen your physician and ruled out non-musculoskeletal causes, this simple and logical program will produce results if you remain patient and stick with it.

▶ **Frequency is more important than quantity.**

Although a certain quantity of work is needed to counterbalance and correct any distortion, three hours once a week is never as good as one hour three times a week or a half hour six times a week. When there's a particular problem distortion that's causing a lot of pain and needs additional special attention, 15 minutes twice a day is good, 10 minutes three times a day is better. Obviously, you'll need to adapt your pain relief program to your life and schedule, and that's great; just do the best you can to keep a steady input of corrective stretching and exercise coming into your body to counteract the steady daily input of pain-causing postural distortion.

▶ **For as long as your daily work or lifestyle uses some muscles more than others, you will *always* have an unbalanced workout if you want to stay out of pain.**

When I said earlier that "your workout can become balanced when your posture becomes balanced, but not until then," that was true. If, however, after you become posturally balanced, you continue to engage in those daily activities and assume those habitual postures that created the distortion in the first place and caused your pain, you will continue to need a workout that is unbalanced enough in the opposite direction to keep your posture balanced. In the case of the chest muscles, suppose you get the chest and back muscles balanced and the shoulders become correctly aligned posturally. If, thereafter, you continue to work at your computer for eight hours a day each day, your chest muscles will soon adaptively shorten again unless your workout remains unbalanced enough in the opposite direction to counteract your daily "desk workout."

▶ **Your level of commitment and personal responsibility will determine your success.**

It's hard to imagine anyone with pain saying that he or she doesn't want to get rid of that pain, yet when people in pain are shown how they can keep themselves healthy and pain-free, many of them say that it's too much trouble or that they just don't have the time. Such comments are simply indicators of their level of commitment to their own health and pain relief, and typically many of these people will instead seek a quick fix in the form of pain-relieving medications, only to discover, many years later, that their pain is no better and that all the years of taking those medications and neglecting proper self-care have caused them additional, and often worse, problems. If you know that you, and only you, are responsible for your health and pain relief, and if you're willing to move heaven and earth, if that's what it takes, to obtain vibrant, pain-free health, you have what it takes to succeed. (If in doubt, please reread the Introduction, especially the section entitled "Philosophy 101.")

Using the Stretching and Exercise Chapters

The following chapters show you how to select the proper stretches and exercises to correct your postural distortions and reduce or eliminate your pain. In order to make these pages simple to use, the chapters are arranged by body areas and the stretches and exercises are listed under the distortion for which they are to be used as a correction. Here's what you'll find for each distortion:

▶ **Distortion Name.**

▶ **Chart Pattern.**

This is an icon, a small illustration showing what the distortion looks like when properly marked on a chart. This makes it easy to select stretches and exercises for your personal program by giving you a quick visual reference to confirm that you are choosing correctly. If the Chart Pattern icon shown matches the distortion marked on your chart, just add the suggested stretches and exercises to your personal program and you're on your way.

▶ **Goal.**

The goal is a brief summary of what you will be trying to achieve by doing these suggested stretches and exercises. In addition, this section will tell you what to do if the measurement of this particular distortion was unclear for some reason. However, it is vitally important to remember one thing: The goal, as well as the rules given and the suggestions made regarding what to stretch and strengthen, apply *only* during the time when you are trying to correct for that particular distortion. Once that distortion has been corrected and, assuming you are not continuing to engage in activities that would tend to make it return, the rules for creating an unbalanced corrective workout no longer apply and you can stretch and strengthen the opposing muscle groups equally. If the distortion starts to come back, however, the unbalanced workout rules apply once again until that distortion is gone.

▶ **What to Stretch.**
 Which muscles or areas to stretch.

▶ **What to Strengthen.**
 Which muscles or areas to strengthen.

▶ **Suggestion(s) for Stretching.**
 One or more suggested stretches to help correct the distortion.

▶ **Suggestion(s) for Strengthening.**
 One or more suggested strengthening exercises to help correct the distortion.

▶ **Notes and Contraindications.**
 This section will appear as necessary in order to give you additional information or to warn you of any contraindications or things to watch out for or be aware of. Always check for and read any notes and contraindications listed before you begin using the related stretches or exercises in your program.

For every muscle or muscle group in the body there are many different stretches and exercises possible. Indeed, you may already have your favorites, and if not, there are many good books available on exercise and stretching. Accordingly, the presentation of certain stretches and exercises in the following chapters is in no way meant to imply that you cannot or should not try using others; they are simply some that I have found very helpful and easy for people to learn and use. If you have other stretches or exercises that you prefer, by all means feel free to use them instead of, or in addition to, those shown here. **Caution:** Make *very sure*, however, that they in fact accomplish the goal listed for each distortion and are not actually working against you. It is both foolish and frustrating to spend weeks or months diligently following a workout program, only to find out that the stretches and exercises you're using have actually been making your problem worse. If in doubt, just use the ones shown in this book.

One additional note should be added here. Although the rest of the chapters in this section deal with postural corrections for various parts of the body, you'll notice that none of the chapter headings specifically mention the back. This is not an oversight, but rather a reflection of the fact that in the process of using the corrective stretches and exercises given for the pelvis, shoulders, and neck, you will be making the necessary corrections for the back.

Of Reps, Sets, and Such

As you will see when you start to choose the stretches and exercises for your personal program, no quantities are given for the number of repetitions or sets to do or the amount of weight or resistance to use. This is deliberate, as it is impossible to give specific recommendations in a book intended for a diverse audience; after all, what would be appropriate for a competitive athlete in his or her prime would almost certainly be inappropriate, or even potentially harmful, for a sedentary, middle-aged office worker. As with choosing the proper stretches and exercises to correct your individual distortions and relieve your specific pain, it is important that you likewise tailor the frequency, quantity, difficulty, and duration of each stretch or exercise to your individual needs, capacity, and level of fitness. Accordingly, here are a few basic guidelines:

1. If tackling all your postural distortions at once seems too daunting, begin with the larger or more important distortions—the ones that cause you the most pain—and gradually add corrections for the less important ones as you develop your personal program. For example, if you have low back and neck pain and your pelvis is very anteriorly rotated, it's far more important to correct the anterior pelvic rotation than to worry about correcting your slightly pronated forearms. However, if your major pain complaint is forearm, wrist, and hand pain and your forearms are severely pronated, it makes more sense to focus your pain relief program first on correcting your forearm pronation.

2. When stretching, *never* force anything; stretch gently and easily, giving your muscles time to adapt to the new demands you're placing on them. Also, *never* "bounce" in a stretch; find a point where you feel a good, steady, comfortable stretch, then hold it at that level. If you find during the stretch that the muscles loosen up and you can do a little more, slightly increase the range and/or duration of the stretch.

3. How long should you hold a stretch and how many should you do? There are several theories of stretching, each with a slightly different idea on stretch technique, duration, and quantity, so if you have a system that works for you, by all means use it. I've found that a steady stretch of 15 to 30 seconds seems to give the best results in most cases, the quantity is dependent on the current condition of your muscles and whether an increased number of repetitions gives you increased flexibility. If five repetitions get you no more flexibility than three, do only three. Remember, too, as noted previously, that frequency is more important than quantity.

4. When doing strengthening exercises, always start slowly, especially if you have areas of major pain, using fewer repetitions, less time, and/or less weight than you think you can handle. It's easy to build up later if you find your initial program too easy, but it's frustrating and painful to injure yourself and make yourself worse by attempting too much too soon. If you are going to use weights or exercise machines at a gym or health club and are unfamiliar with their proper use, always get qualified instruction so that you can exercise safely and avoid creating more pain for yourself.

5. A good rule of thumb for strength training is to start with one set of eight to 12 repetitions, using about 70 to 80 percent of the maximum amount of resistance you can handle. When doing 12 repetitions at that weight becomes quite easy, try increasing the resistance no more than about 5 percent and building up again from eight repetitions to 12 repetitions. Additional sets of similar numbers of repetitions can be added as necessary, perhaps by exercising those muscles more frequently, to counterbalance postural distortions and increase the corrective effect.

A Last Reminder

I know I've already said this in the Preface, but it bears repeating here, as you prepare to start creating your pain relief program:

This book is not intended to provide medical advice or to diagnose or treat any medical condition. The exercises, stretches, ideas, and recommendations presented are those that I have found helpful and effective in restoring proper muscular balance, creating good postural alignment, and reducing or eliminating pain. However, although they are time tested, based on common sense and sound principles, and have worked for many people, they may not be appropriate for you or your particular condition. Accordingly, it is recommended that you obtain the approval of your physician or other primary healthcare provider before beginning this or any exercise or stretching program. Also, there are other causes of pain, such as injury and disease, that are not within the scope of this book and may require other forms of treatment. These conditions should be ruled out by your physician or other primary healthcare provider before you begin this program.

Chapter 11

Skeletal Asymmetries:
Fixing the Foundation First

At 15, when his mother first brought him to see me, Brett had already experienced several years of chronic neck pain. His family physician, a chiropractor, and a neurologist had all examined him but had found nothing wrong, no reason why his neck should be hurting him so badly. After performing a postural examination, I explained to Brett that his left leg appeared to be about 5/16-inch shorter than his right and that such a leg length difference could well be the root cause of his neck pain. Brett was eager to try a 5/16-inch lift in his left shoe if that would help get rid of his pain, and once he started wearing the lift his neck pain began to ease within a day or two, was gone within two weeks, and has not returned in the three years since.

If you have cracks in the walls of your house and want to repair them, it is important first to make sure the foundation is level and solid before making the repairs; otherwise, if your foundation is tilted or unstable, the house will sooner or later shift again, the cracks will recur, and you'll end up having to repair the same cracks time after time. The same principle applies to your body. If your leg lengths are unequal, your pelvis is supported by two columns of bone of different lengths, causing the pelvis to tilt downward on the side of the shorter leg and forcing a variety of muscles throughout the body to contract continuously to compensate. Even if your legs are the same length, if the two halves of your pelvis are unequal, the same type of tilting to the smaller side will occur, especially when sitting, resulting in the same type of muscular compensation. If you don't want to keep fixing your body's pain problems time after time, it only makes sense to be sure that your foundation is level first.

After doing hundreds and hundreds of postural evaluations of people in pain, I am convinced that the failure to recognize and to correct for skeletal asymmetries is a major reason why so many techniques and treatments fail to provide lasting, long-term musculoskeletal pain relief. Even if a particular treatment or medication provides short-term relief, if it has to be repeated week after week, month after month, and year after year, there is a missing piece, a root cause that needs to be addressed. No matter how skilled any physician or therapist may be, if you get off the treatment table—mine or anyone else's—and go right back to standing and/or sitting with a tilted pelvis, your muscles will once again tighten up to compensate, and any pain they were causing before will return. I know; my muscles did exactly that for nearly 30 years, from my early teens to my early 40s, until after I had gotten into this profession, discovered my leg length inequality, and figured out how to correct for it.

I have also seen a clear distinction between those clients with skeletal asymmetries who correct for them and those who don't. As a group, those who correct for their asymmetries and stand, walk, and sit with a level pelvis generally reduce or eliminate their pain more quickly and more lastingly, whereas those who elect not to make corrections often make little or no progress and typically complain of many of the same pains even after weeks in treatment. Perhaps most revealing are the cases of those who, after not correcting for their skeletal asymmetries, finally decide to give it a try, only to find, often much to their surprise, that their pain starts to decrease and they begin to feel better. To put it simply, if all the readers of this book who have musculoskeletal pain were to do nothing else in this program but to simply measure and correct for any skeletal asymmetries, I suspect that a majority of them would experience a noticeable, and in many cases significant, reduction in their chronic pain.

Leg Length Inequality (LLI)

The ideal way to measure LLI is with a standing X-ray, preferably with a special extra-long film cassette that can take a picture from the top of the pelvis to the ankles in all but the tallest individuals. This allows the full length of the upper and lower leg bones to be seen and measured directly on the film in order to determine if a length difference exists. Unfortunately, X-ray machines with this kind of large cassette are usually found only in hospitals and orthopedic or sports medicine clinics, so they may or may not be readily available to you and your doctor.

It is also possible to use a regular X-ray machine with a standard size cassette to take a picture of only the pelvis, including the heads of the femurs or thigh bones, and to note on the film the difference in height of the femoral heads (the tops of the two thigh bones). However, this requires extremely precise positioning of the patient by the X-ray technician, and even an apparently minor error can render the X-ray measurement useless. As an example, let's assume that the technician fails to note that the arch in your right foot has fallen more than the left, or that, although you're standing with your left knee straight, your right knee is slightly buckled. In either case, the top of the right femur will appear lower than it otherwise would, making the measurement inaccurate and meaningless. This is why being able to measure the full length of the bones on an extra-long X-ray film that shows both ends of the bones is so desirable. Although MRI (magnetic resonance imaging) is also an excellent method of LLI evaluation, its cost typically is significantly greater and access to an MRI center may be limited in certain areas.

However, appropriate X-ray facilities may not be available in all areas, or you simply may prefer not to be x-rayed unless absolutely necessary, so it's nice to know that there is a simple way for you and a partner to try to estimate your leg length differences. Although you must always bear in mind that it is only an estimate, rather than a precise measurement, it's surprising how accurate a trained and experienced examiner can become with this method.

The first thing to do is to look on your partner's postural chart at the measurements you took at the pelvis. Assuming you took the measurements accurately and in accordance with the procedures given earlier, if the lines at the greater trochanters on both the front and back views are level, the legs should be equal in length and there's no need to check for a LLI. However, use the procedure outlined in "Estimating Leg Length Inequalities (see page 124) if one or more of the following conditions apply:

▶ Those lines were slanted, indicating that one trochanter appeared lower.

▶ The two trochanter lines don't agree.

▶ You're just feeling unsure and want to recheck your measurements.

In order to estimate the leg length difference, you will first need to have on hand shims of different thickness, as follows: 1/8", 3/16", 1/4", 5/16", 3/8". (A shim is a piece of material, such as wood, metal, cork, or rubber, placed under one side or one corner of a structure or piece of equipment to level it—for example, a matchbook or folded napkin put under the leg of a tippy table.) This covers the range of leg length discrepancies that I most commonly find, although they are smaller than most doctors think is significant. If the difference you're measuring is somewhat larger, these shims can be combined into a range of thickness up to 1-1/4", although by this point you're looking at a difference that you would certainly know about already. Although I use special shim material of measured thickness in my office, there's no need to rush out and buy anything special when you can easily improvise by using some magazines and a ruler. Get a stack of old magazines of various thickness and measure them to see if any of them exactly match one of the dimensions listed; if so, mark the thickness on it and set it aside. When measuring, be sure to squeeze the edges of the pages tightly together, as they would be with someone standing on them. If a magazine is slightly too thick, simply cut out or tear out pages until the thickness is correct; if no magazine is thick enough for the larger sizes, simply combine two or more thinner magazines and staple some of their pages together so that they form a single, thicker shim.

Estimating Leg Length Inequalities

Now that you have your shims made, you're ready to begin. Here's a step by-step method for estimating LLI:

1. If the arches of the feet are equal, this procedure is best done with your partner in bare feet, although shoes of equal height (no lifts or supports in one shoe that are not in the other) may be worn, if necessary. However, if the arches of the feet are unequal, your partner must stand either on good orthotics that equalize the arches or in shoes of equal height with good and equal arch supports.

2. Throughout this process, make sure that your partner stands with the feet no more than about 3 to 4 inches apart and both knees straight (not flexed or hyperextended). If your partner is laterally rotated at the pelvis, with one side of the pelvis more anterior than the other, turn the pelvis back so that the pelvis is even, with neither side anterior. Instruct your partner to hold this position while you are measuring.

3. Kneeling in front of your partner, measure at the top of the greater trochanters, just as you did when doing the original postural evaluation (see Figure 7-5); then repeat the measurement from the back (see Figure 8-3). If the trochanters appear level from both the front and the back, the legs should be equal. If the trochanters are not level, go on to step 4.

4. Using a full-foot shim of known thickness, have your partner stand with the foot of the apparently shorter leg on the shim. Repeat the trochanter measurements, as in Step 3. If the trochanters now appear level from both the front and the back, the shim is correct and the thickness of the shim is the approximate amount of the LLI. If the trochanters are not level, repeat the process, using thicker or thinner shims, until the trochanters level out. Always be sure to correct any pelvic rotation and/or knee flexion or hyperextension each time before measuring in order to help avoid error and make the estimate as accurate as possible.

Notes and Contraindications

1. Always remember that this is *only* an estimate and *not* an exact measurement. Only a medical doctor, osteopath, or chiropractor can give an exact measurement of leg length inequality, so if you suspect a leg length inequality you should have it confirmed by your physician.

2. In my experience, it is much better to use a full-foot lift and **not** a heel lift. A heel lift causes the pelvis on the lifted side to shift forward, resulting in a lateral rotation of the pelvis toward the opposite side, whereas a full-foot lift simply lifts the whole foot straight up without causing any additional distortion. To experience the difference in your own body, even if your legs are equal, stand with one heel—not the whole foot, just the heel—on the end of one of the thicker full-foot shims, say 3/8", and let your body settle as it will. If you've done this correctly, you should feel your pelvis swing forward on the heel lift side and around toward the other side. Now try it again, but this time put the shim under the whole foot; it should lift you straight up on the shim side but not make you sway forward the way the heel lift did. Because the whole purpose here is to eliminate postural distortion and reduce pain, why would you want to create an additional postural distortion that will then have to be corrected and that can also result in additional pain?

3. If you suspect you have a LLI, the first step is to get it measured as accurately as possible, ideally by a physician's X-ray. Once you know the actual difference, the second step is to test a full-foot lift of that thickness in a loose-fitting shoe (perhaps an athletic shoe) in order to make sure that your body agrees. If, after wearing the lift for perhaps a week or two, it feels good, helps to balance you out, and relieves your pain, you're all set for step 3: having the lift added to the sole of your shoe by a shoe repair store (For more on this, see "Correcting Shoes," later in this chapter).

4. Although it is not common, it is possible that an occasional individual may have a wedge-shaped vertebra, such that when looked at from the front or back the body of the vertebra is not as tall (thick) on one side as it is on the other. This causes the vertebra above it to sit at an angle, resulting in a tilted spinal column above the wedge-shaped vertebra and consequent muscular compensation. A similar effect, also relatively uncommon, can be produced by a sacrum that is misaligned (that is, tilted to one side) within the pelvis itself. If you feel certain that one leg is short, yet adding a lift under that leg to equalize the leg lengths causes increased pain, remove the lift and contact your physician for an evaluation.

Small Hemipelvis

As with LLI, the only absolutely precise way to verify the existence and amount of a small hemipelvis is with an X-ray of the pelvis or some other similarly accurate imaging procedure. However, it is possible, using the shims you created to measure LLI, to check for the possible existence of a small hemipelvis and to estimate the approximate correction needed.

Checking for a Small Hemipelvis

1. To check for a small hemipelvis, have your partner sit on a hard, level surface, such as a desk, table, counter, or bench. Your partner's feet should be supported high enough that there is a slight air space or gap between the front edge of the surface and the backs of your partner's thighs. Instruct your partner to sit absolutely upright, with the spine perfectly vertical, during the measurements.

2. Take a measurement at the iliac crest, just as you did in the standing measurements from the front (see Figure 7-4), to determine if one side is higher than the other. Remember to kneel or squat to bring your eyes to the level of your measurement. If one side is lower, suspect a small hemipelvis on that side.

3. To estimate the correction needed, have your partner sit with a shim of known thickness under the ischial tuberosity or "sitzbone" at the bottom of the pelvis on the shorter side. As you did when doing the postural evaluation, take a measurement at the iliac crests, the top edges of the pelvis. If necessary, remeasure using different shims until the iliac crests seem approximately level. Have your partner sit on the chosen shim for a few minutes, then remove the shim and let your partner sit without it and notice the difference. You can repeat this process as needed until your partner gets a sense of whether the shim feels correct, but ultimately the best test is simply to use the shim or lift for a few days during any extended periods of sitting. If sitting on a lift helps to relax the muscles, eases pain, and/or makes it easier to sit comfortably for longer periods without fidgeting, the chances are that the lift is either correct or very nearly so. As always, remember that only a physician can officially diagnose and precisely measure the amount of any structural asymmetries.

4. Once the correct lift thickness to be used under the ischial tuberosity has been determined, a correction of roughly one-half that thickness is generally needed under the full foot on that side if—but only if—the leg lengths are equal. If, in addition to the small hemipelvis, a leg length inequality exists, the situation is more com-

plex than is appropriate to deal with in a book like this and you should refer the matter to a physician or other trained evaluator.

Notes and Contraindications

1. Always remember that this is *only* an estimate and *not* an exact measurement. Only a medical doctor, osteopath, or chiropractor can give you an exact measurement of any structural asymmetry, so if you suspect a small hemipelvis you should have it confirmed by your physician.

2. If a small hemipelvis does in fact exist, it is vitally important to correct it, even if the amount of correction seems trivial. The relief brought by even a small correction can sometimes be life-changing, and it can often be the missing piece that has frustrated earlier efforts at pain relief.

3. The measurement is taken with your partner sitting on a hard surface to ensure the most accurate possible estimate of the difference. However, the lift thickness used under the ischial tuberosity when sitting on a hard surface should be approximately doubled when sitting on a somewhat padded surface, such as an office chair or car seat, and should be approximately tripled when sitting on a very soft surface, such as an overstuffed couch.[1]

4. As mentioned in the discussion of leg length inequality, it is possible that an occasional individual may have a wedge-shaped vertebra, such that when looked at from the front or back the body of the vertebra is not as tall (thick) on one side as it is on the other. This causes the vertebra above it to sit at an angle, resulting in a tilted spinal column above the wedge-shaped vertebra and consequent muscular compensation. A similar effect, also relatively uncommon, can be produced by a sacrum that is misaligned (that is, tilted to one side) within the pelvis itself. If you feel certain that one hemipelvis is smaller, yet adding a shim under that ischial tuberosity ("sitzbone") to level the pelvis causes increased pain, remove the shim and contact your physician for an evaluation.

Tilted Arches

Each foot has three arches, but the one you measured is the medial longitudinal arch, which runs from the front of the heel to the base of the big toe and, when normal, bows the inside edge of the foot up off the floor. If that arch is bowed too high, the foot and ankle tend to roll outward and ride on the outer edge of the foot (inversion or supination). A more common distortion, however, is eversion or pronation, in which the arch collapses, either partially or totally, and the foot and ankle tend to roll inward toward the midline of the body. Because the feet are the foundation on which the rest of the body stands, having a tilted foundation will obviously cause tilting and muscular compensation in the rest of the body, often with resultant tension and pain.

Although exercises can be very beneficial in correcting some distortions of the feet and ankle, the use of foot orthotics (corrective arch supports) is often helpful and sometimes necessary. A detailed discussion of orthotics, however, is beyond the scope of this book, so if your measurements indicate a marked inward or outward tilt at the ankle, you should seek the advice of a trained professional to see if orthotics might be helpful in correcting the condition and reducing pain. If you already have orthotics and want to test to see if they are about right for you, stand in bare feet on your orthotics with your feet about 3 to 4 inches apart and pointing straight ahead, then do a slight knee bend. If your orthotics are right for you, the center of your kneecap on each side should track forward right over the second toe of the corresponding foot. If your kneecap tracks more toward the inside or outside of your foot, you may need new orthotics or an adjustment to your old ones. This test can be helpful as a rough guide, but in case of doubt always consult a properly trained healthcare practitioner for a complete orthotic evaluation.

If you're having a lot of foot problems or foot pain, you might want to consult a podiatrist, whereas if your pain is mostly elsewhere, many chiropractors or orthopedic specialists also prescribe orthotics and can perhaps give you a broader range of evaluation and other treatment, if necessary. Pre-molded arch supports are available at some sporting goods stores or stores that specialize in sports shoes and, although they may sometimes solve the problem, I normally recommend that people get custom-fitted orthotics. They don't cost that much more, and if you have significant foot or postural problems it's usually well worth it, especially when you consider that you're typically getting a doctor's supervision for that price. Trying to cut costs on your body's foundation is like trying to cut costs on the foundation of your new house; naturally, you don't want to overpay, but using top-quality materials under the supervision of a qualified contractor will give you a reliable foundation that will really last.

One further note: In my experience, podiatrists tend to prescribe harder, more rigid orthotics, and their prices generally include evaluation and any required follow-up care. Chiropractors, on the other hand, generally seem to favor softer, somewhat flexible orthotics, and they, too, usually include their evaluation and any follow-up adjustments to the orthotics in their pricing. Both types of orthotics have their advocates, but you're the one who's going to be wearing them, so ask your orthotics provider why he or she favors a particular kind, and also be sure to ask to try standing on a sample pair, if available. Although they won't be custom-molded for your feet, they will at least give you an idea before you buy of what wearing that type might be like. Also, be sure to shop around; you may be surprised at how prices, orthotic types, and levels of service can vary.

Dealing With Skeletal Asymmetries

As noted in the beginning of this chapter and also in Chapter 4, the correction of skeletal asymmetries is vitally important if you want to achieve pain relief for life. Here is a summary of some basic principles to keep in mind:

▸ Remember: Any apparent skeletal differences you've found are only estimates. The techniques discussed in this chapter for estimating the amount of LLI or a small hemipelvis are necessarily modified versions of those I use and teach, because more advanced estimating techniques require hands-on instruction and supervision to learn properly, and even those more advanced techniques are still only estimates. The only way to get an exact measurement of these kinds of asymmetries is to have them measured on film by a physician.

▸ Because you are in charge of your own body, you are always free to experiment with putting different lifts under your foot and/or pelvis to see what it feels like to stand, walk, or sit that way. If the lift makes you feel better, it's probably helpful for you; if it makes you feel worse, it may be wrong for you, so take it out. However, always tell your physician what you intend to do and ask if there is any medical reason why you shouldn't try leveling your pelvis this way; even if your physician chooses not to x-ray you to measure the difference(s) exactly, if he or she knows of no reason why you shouldn't experiment, you can do so with confidence.

▸ Although only a physician can exactly measure skeletal differences, only **you** get to decide whether correcting them is important. Although a physician or other evaluator may tell you that your 3/16-inch leg length difference or 1/8-inch smaller hemipelvis is "insignificant" or "not enough to be important," remember the quotations from doctors Travell and Simons in Chapter 4 (see page 49) about the importance of correcting leg length inequalities as small as 1/8 inch in order to achieve pain relief. You, and only you, ultimately get to decide whether such corrections are or are not important to your body, because only you live in your body and only you know what it feels like to stand, walk, and/or sit with and without the lift(s). Although it's always important to listen to the advice of a good physician, it is equally important to listen to the advice of your body if you really want to achieve effective pain relief.

▶ If you've confirmed that you do indeed have a difference in leg length or hemipelvis size, and if using a lift helps to reduce or eliminate your pain, it's important to correct for the difference at all times. If you need a lift under your foot to keep your pelvis level, you should try not to walk barefoot unless absolutely necessary, because that will cause the pelvis to tilt, thereby restarting the chain of muscular compensation and, ultimately, pain. Obviously some common sense comes into play here; if you get up in the middle of the night to go to the bathroom, no, it's not critical for that brief trip that you put on shoes or slippers that have been leveled up. I often explain it to clients by saying that if I'm sitting in a chair at home in the summer with my shoes kicked off and I get up to get a glass of water, I usually don't bother to put on my shoes for the one minute I'm going to be up, but if I'm getting up to fix dinner or do some work around the house, I put them on to keep my pelvis level. It all boils down to this, really: The more time you spend standing or sitting with a tilted pelvis, the more your muscles will have to compensate and the more pain you'll have; the more time you spend standing or sitting with a level pelvis, the more your muscles can relax and the less pain you'll have. As we discussed in the Introduction, it's your body and your pain, so it's your choice.

▶ Please understand: I am **not** suggesting that every reader of this book, no matter how pain-free, absolutely must correct any or all skeletal asymmetries. This book is intended to help those in pain, though it will also help those without pain to stay that way. If you discover that you have a small leg length or pelvic asymmetry but you're blissfully pain-free, it's probably not important that you rush out and correct the asymmetry immediately, although it's good to know about it in case you start to develop painful symptoms in the future. However, even if you're pain-free, if your job requires maximum physical strength and flexibility, as well as optimum, injury-free performance—for example, as an athlete, dancer, police officer, firefighter, or military officer—you might want to try to correct for even relatively small skeletal asymmetries and see how it affects your physical performance, strength, and balance. Either way, it's up to you; it's your body, so you get to make the decisions.

Correcting Shoes

Once you've established that you do in fact have a leg length or hemipelvis difference, you'll want to see how it feels to stand and walk level. Experimenting with a full-foot lift inside your shoe to see what thickness you need is fine as a temporary measure, but getting a full-foot lift and your foot into a tight shoe can sometimes be a problem and is usually not the best long-term solution. The toe box on any shoe (the front portion of the shoe where your toes fit) only has just so much room in it, so when you add a lift, especially a thick lift, under your foot inside the shoe, it may push your toes up against the top of the shoe and cramp them, making the shoe difficult or impossible to wear. As a result, the ideal method of correction, whenever possible, is to have the required thickness added by a cobbler to the sole of the shoe from heel to toe, a procedure that can be done relatively inexpensively and unobtrusively, thus keeping the correction out of the foot compartment. Please note, though, that not all shoes can be easily corrected externally, so if it's difficult or impossible to add an external lift in the sole of certain shoes, as for example in athletic shoes that have air or gel bladders in their soles, you may still need to use an internal full-foot lift in those shoes as a long-term solution. If you have any questions about which kinds of shoes can or can't be adjusted, talk to a good shoe-repair technician, preferably one who has had a lot of experience in making these kinds of full-foot corrections. I can tell you from experience that not all shoe-repair shops are good at this, so it's worth looking around until you find someone really skilled and experienced.

In any case, it's always a good idea to experiment with an internal lift first, perhaps finding some loose pair of shoes, sandals, or boots into which the lift will fit, so that you can test whether the amount of correction offered by the lift feels right to you. After all, there's no sense in running out and having all your shoes adjusted only to discover that you need a little more correction or a little less, so testing first with a lift in your shoe only makes good sense. You can usually obtain a piece of acceptable material, such as rubber or orthopedic crepe, from your local shoe repair store. The only requirements are that the material be of the correct thickness, firm enough to hold that thickness under your body weight, able to conform to the inside of the shoe, resistant to moisture, and reasonably comfortable under your foot. Just place the material on the floor, stand on it with your bare foot, trace around your foot with a pen, and then cut out the outline of your foot and trim it as needed to fit in the bottom of your shoe.

If you have no choice but to use internal lifts long-term in certain types of shoes, you can try to buy those shoes slightly larger or wider to allow more room in the toe box for the lift. One good idea is to take your internal lift to the shoe store and insert it into the new shoe before trying it on. Remember also that you can often create more room for the lift in the toe box of athletic shoes (and some casual shoes) by removing the arch supports or liners from the inside of the shoes. Be very sure, however, that you either remove the liners from *both* shoes or leave them both in. If you only take out the liner on the lift side, the thickness of the liner in the other shoe will decrease the net amount of correction of the lift. Just remember that, although the lift only goes in the shoe with the shorter leg, everything else should be done equally (that is, both liners or none, two orthotics or none, and so on). That way, the net difference between the two shoes will always be the thickness of the lift. Also, if the full-foot lift is thin enough, or the shoes are roomy enough, that you can leave the liners in, be sure to stick the lift under the shoe liner so that you can get the benefit of the arch support and cushioning that the shoe liner offers.

Although most bodies adapt quickly to a correct lift, it occasionally happens that some people experience brief twinges of discomfort while their muscles are adapting to their new alignment, but this discomfort usually disappears fairly quickly. If, however, this discomfort persists, or if wearing the lift in the shoe causes real pain, the lift should be removed at once. First of all, double check to make sure that it is the correct thickness and that it is in fact being used under the correct foot. (If you put it under the longer leg, your body will let you know right away!) If all that is correct, try to introduce the lift gradually, starting perhaps by wearing it for one hour at a time, then for two hours, for four hours, for six hours, and so on. If the discomfort still persists but you are confident that the lift thickness is correct, it may be advisable to try a lift of perhaps half of the required thickness for a while, then, once the body is used to that, to progress (by stages, if necessary) to using a lift of the full thickness. If even this gradual approach still produces discomfort, remove the lift and seek the advice of your physician.

At this point, I can hear the anguished cries of some readers who suffer from what I call "Imelda Marcos Syndrome," named after the shoe-collecting wife of the late Philippine ruler Ferdinand Marcos: "Do you know how many pairs of shoes I have? It'll cost me a fortune to have them all corrected!" Well, let's address this and try to bring those of you with lots of shoes a little peace and comfort. You don't have to correct all your shoes at once; simply start with the shoes you wear the most, then gradually work your way down to those you rarely wear. Assuming you've confirmed and are using the proper thickness in your shoes, once you get used to walking and standing level, the pain relief and comfort you'll experience should provide more than enough motivation for you to go ahead and correct the less-used shoes, or else to get rid of them if they're simply not important enough to correct. Besides, if you think correcting a few shoes is expensive, how expensive is it to have pain—the doctor visits, medications, perhaps even hospitalizations, surgeries, and lost income from absence at work? Do you see what I mean? I've always found that staying pain-free and in good health is much less expensive (and far more enjoyable!) than waiting until I get pain or illness and then having to fight my way back to health. Still, as I've emphasized so many times, it's your body, so it's your choice; choose well!

Chapter 12

Standing Firm:
Aligning the
Feet and Ankles

Juan had deep, aching pain in his right upper back and shoulder, but worst of all was the pain that radiated down his right arm and into his wrist and hand. After a medical evaluation that revealed no injuries or problems in his cervical spine, he had been sent home with a prescription for pain relievers. I did a postural evaluation that showed both a collapsed arch in his left foot and a slightly shorter left leg, a combination that caused the left side of Juan's pelvis and his left shoulder to drop, which in turn caused the muscles on the right side of his neck to stay in constant contraction in order to hold his head upright. This was the confirmation we needed, because his pain pattern matched that of the scalene muscles of the neck.

After relieving the trigger points in his right scalene muscles that were causing his pain, I referred Juan for orthotics to equalize the arches in his feet and for some material to experiment with in his shoe to level his pelvis and raise his left shoulder. I also suggested some stretches and home therapy to keep his right scalene muscles relaxed, then explained that as long as he wore his orthotics and his foot lift in his left shoe his shoulders should remain level and his pain should not return. Although Juan was surprised that supporting his feet would keep his arm pain at bay, he followed the program and his pain has not come back.

Distortion: Dropped/Flattened Arches

Chart Pattern

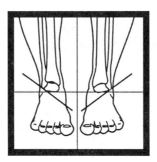

Goal

If the arches have dropped or flattened, the feet are everted or pronated and the muscles that cause pronation are shortened and tight, whereas the muscles that cause the opposite condition, inversion or supination, are stretched and weak. With flattened arches, the ankles tend to roll inward and downward, so the goal here is to strengthen the opposing muscles that roll the ankles outward and upward. Remember that if one arch is flattened but the other one is normal, only do these stretches and exercises on the side with the flattened arch. If the measurement is unclear on either arch, do a balanced workout of that foot and ankle unless further evaluation gives a clear indication of distortion.

What to Stretch

▶ Muscles that turn the sole of the foot outward (everters or pronators); see Figure 12-1.

What to Strengthen

▶ Muscles that turn the sole of the foot inward (inverters or supinators); see Figure 12-1.

Suggestion(s) for Stretching

Sit with your fist held between your knees as shown in Figure 12-1. Lift up the inside edges of the feet while keeping the outer edges on the floor.

Suggestion(s) for Strengthening

Same as "Suggestions for Stretching." For variety, you can sit with bare feet 6 inches apart on a towel, then keeping the heels still, gather the towel medially (toward the space between your feet) with the toes.

Notes and Contraindications

▶ Reminder: If the flattening of the arches is very marked or severe, you should consult a trained healthcare professional to see if orthotics might be helpful in correcting the condition and reducing pain.

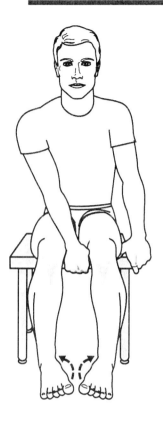

Figure 12-1

Distortion: High Arches

Chart Pattern

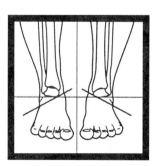

Goal

If the arches are too high, the feet are inverted or supinated and the muscles that cause supination are shortened and tight, whereas the muscles that cause the opposite condition, eversion or pronation, are stretched and weak. With high arches, the ankles tend to roll outward and upward, so the goal here is to strengthen the opposing muscles that roll the ankles inward and downward. Remember that if one arch is high but the other one is normal,

137

only do these stretches and exercises on the side with the high arch. If the measurement is unclear on either arch, do a balanced workout of that foot and ankle unless further evaluation gives a clear indication of distortion.

What to Stretch

▶ Muscles that turn the sole of the foot inward (inverters or supinators); see Figure 12-2.

What to Strengthen

▶ Muscles that turn the sole of the foot outward (everters or pronators); see Figure 12-2.

Suggestion(s) for Stretching

Sit with your fist held between your knees as shown in Figure 12-2. Lift up the outside edges of the feet while keeping the inside edges on the floor.

Suggestion(s) for Strengthening

Same as "Suggestions for Stretching."

Notes and Contraindications

▶ Reminder: If the high arches are very marked or severe, you should consult a trained healthcare professional to see if orthotics might be helpful in correcting the condition and reducing pain.

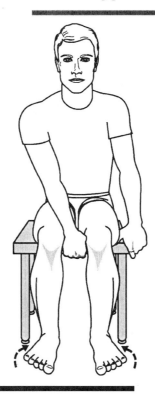

Figure 12-2

Distortion: Feet Laterally Rotated

Chart Pattern

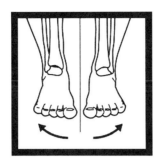

Goal

The feet should be pointing essentially forward when standing. If either foot is laterally rotated, it is caused by lateral rotation of the leg at the hip. If the measurement is unclear on either leg, work both lateral and medial hip rotators equally on that leg.

What to Stretch

▶ Hip muscles that turn the leg outward (lateral hip rotators); see Figure 12-3.

What to Strengthen

▶ Hip muscles that turn the leg inward (medial hip rotators); see Figure 12-4.

Suggestion(s) for Stretching

Lie face down as shown in Figure 12-3 with involved leg bent. Keeping pelvis and torso flat on floor, let bent leg rotate outward. Ankle weight is optional.

Suggestion(s) for Strengthening

Sit with anchored exercise tubing or resistance cable looped around ankle of involved leg, as shown. Keeping knees relatively close together, rotate ankle of involved leg outward. If necessary, stabilize knee position by clasping hands around active knee. (See Figure 12-4.)

Notes and Contraindications

▶ When the foot is very laterally rotated, the arch tends to be flattened during walking as the foot rolls from heel strike through mid-stance to toe-off, and the great toe is sometimes pushed laterally during toe-off, which may contribute to the formation of a bunion. If either of these conditions exists, or if the lateral rotation of the foot is marked, it is advisable to seek evaluation for orthotics, as they may give much-needed support while you are working to correct the lateral rotation with this program.

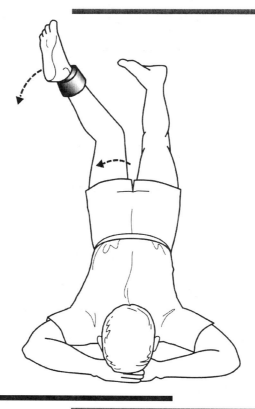

Figure 12-3

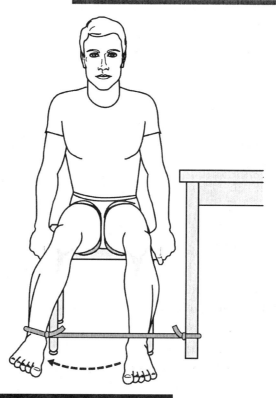

Figure 12-4

Distortion: Feet Medially Rotated

Chart Pattern

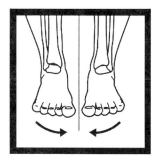

Goal

The feet should be pointing essentially forward when standing. If either foot is medially rotated, it is caused by medial rotation of the leg at the hip. If the measurement is unclear on either leg, work both lateral and medial rotators equally on that leg.

What to Stretch

▶ Hip muscles that turn the leg inward (medial hip rotators); see Figure 12-5.

What to Strengthen

▶ Hip muscles that turn the leg outward (lateral hip rotators); see Figure 12-6.

Suggestion(s) for Stretching

Stand with involved leg on support, as shown in Figure 12-5. Lean forward to increase stretch.

Suggestion(s) for Strengthening

Sit with anchored exercise tubing or resistance cable looped around ankle of involved leg, as shown. Keeping knees relatively close together, rotate ankle of involved leg inward. If necessary, stabilize knee position by clasping hands around active knee. (See Figure 12-6.)

Notes and Contraindications

▶ When the foot is very medially rotated, the ankle tends to roll outward during walking as the foot rolls from heel strike through mid-stance to toe-off, which can sometimes lead to foot problems and/or sprained ankles. If the medial rotation of the foot is marked, it is advisable to seek evaluation for orthotics, as they may give much-needed support while you are working to correct the medial rotation with this program.

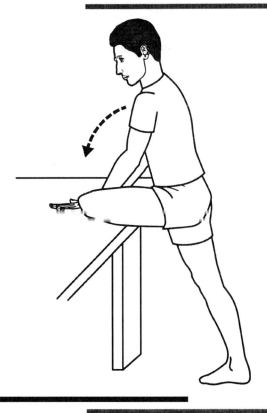

Figure 12-5

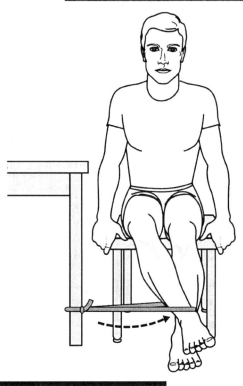

Figure 12-6

Distortion: Ankles Plantar-Flexed

Chart Pattern

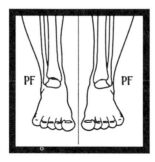

Goal

The plantar surfaces (soles) of the feet should be essentially vertical when you are lying on your back. If the feet point away from the head, it is caused by tight posterior calf muscles. If the measurement is unclear, work both dorsiflexors and plantar flexors (see "What to Stretch" and "What to Strengthen," following) equally, unless you spend a lot of time in high heel shoes or boots. In this case, use a workout slightly unbalanced in the direction of correcting for plantar flexion.

What to Stretch

▶ Muscles that make the ball of your foot push down (plantar flexors); see Figure 12-7 and Figure 12-08.

What to Strengthen

▶ Muscles that pull your foot toward your knee (dorsiflexors); see Figure 12-9.

Suggestion(s) for Stretching

Stand with balls of feet elevated as shown. Bend knees and hold. (See Figure 12-7.)

Sit with towel or belt around involved foot as shown. Pull foot toward you. (See Figure 12-8.)

Suggestion(s) for Strengthening

Pull foot toward knee and hold, as shown in Figure 12-9.

Notes and Contraindications

▶ It is uncommon to find the ankles at rest in dorsiflexion (tops of feet pulled toward the knees). However, if this is the case, simply practice standing or walking on tiptoes, as this strengthens the plantar flexors in the back of the lower leg and stretches the tight dorsiflexors.

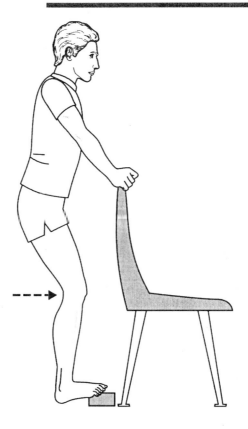

Figure 12-7

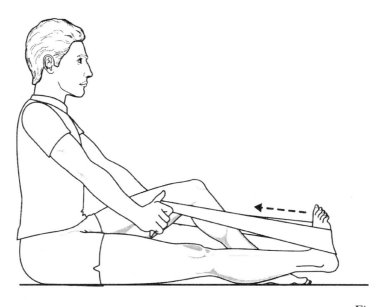

Figure 12-8

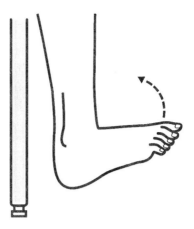

Figure 12-9

Chapter 13

A *Pivotal Issue:*
Keeping the Pelvis Where It Belongs

Paul enjoyed a highly successful career as a financial executive in a major corporation, but he was plagued by almost constant low back tightness and pain, as well as a variety of lesser pain complaints in his head, neck, and shoulders. When a postural evaluation revealed that his pelvis was rotated anteriorly 15 degrees, it was obvious that the last 20 years of sitting at his desk had not been kind to him. I explained to Paul that sitting too much is the scourge of our modern lifestyle, that we were designed to be primarily upright, active beings, and that if he did not begin stretching and exercising the muscles in and around his pelvis, his back pain would only continue to worsen over time, quite possibly leading to one or more operations on his lumbar spine. Desperate to rid himself of the pain that plagued him, Paul readily agreed to do the movement therapy, stretches, and exercises I suggested to release his back muscles and counterbalance the ill effects of his prolonged daily sitting. He worked diligently at his therapy program and within a few weeks found that his back was seldom tight and never painful. "The truth is," he confessed, "I finally realized that it's all up to me. If I do my exercises regularly, my back feels great; if I start to slack off, my back starts to feel the effects of all that sitting and lets me know. The nice thing now is that I know how to keep myself out of pain and it's under my control; all I have to do is actually *do* it!"

In our modern society, because we sit so often and for so long, it is very common for people to be anteriorly rotated in the pelvis, and if so, that should usually be clear when the measurements are taken. However, because the kind of pelvic angle measurement taught in this book—one that can be done without special measuring equipment—is necessarily only a rough approximation, there may well be cases where it is difficult to tell exactly whether the pelvis is rotated anteriorly or posteriorly. If the measurement is unclear, it is generally best to use a relatively balanced workout with a slight emphasis toward correcting anterior (forward) rotation, as this is much more common than posterior pelvic rotation, especially if you spend a lot of time in a seated or hip-flexed position. However, if your lumbar spine (low back) appears flat, rather than having a slight curve forward, do not do the correction for an anterior pelvis, as the pelvis may already be rotated too far posteriorly. Instead, do a moderate, balanced workout until you can get an actual measurement of the pelvic rotation from a trained healthcare professional, then modify your workout if necessary.

Distortion: Lateral Pelvic Tilt

Chart Pattern

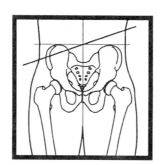

Goal

The pelvis should be level side to side in order to allow the spine to arise vertically from the sacrum. Lateral pelvic tilt, with one side higher than the other, is most frequently the result of a skeletal asymmetry, and any anatomical differences in the bony structure from the bottom of the feet to the top of the pelvis should always be corrected first if lasting results are to be achieved. If the measurement is unclear, work both sides of the body equally unless and until a clear indication of lateral pelvic tilt is found.

What to Stretch

▶ Low side—Muscles that move leg outward (hip abductors); see Figure 13-1.

▶ High side—Muscles that move leg inward (hip adductors); see Figure 13-2.

What to Strengthen

▶ Low side—Muscles that move leg inward (hip adductors); see Figure 13-3.

▶ High side—Muscles that move leg outward (hip abductors); see Figure 13-4.

Suggestion(s) for Stretching

Stand as shown in Figure 13.1 with involved hip toward wall. Press hip toward wall, keeping pelvis and torso erect, and adding pressure with opposite hand, if necessary.

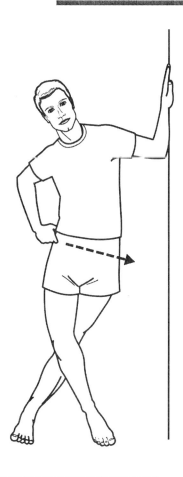

Figure 13-1

Stand with involved leg supported as shown in Figure 13-2. Keeping pelvis upright, lower pelvis while bending standing leg.

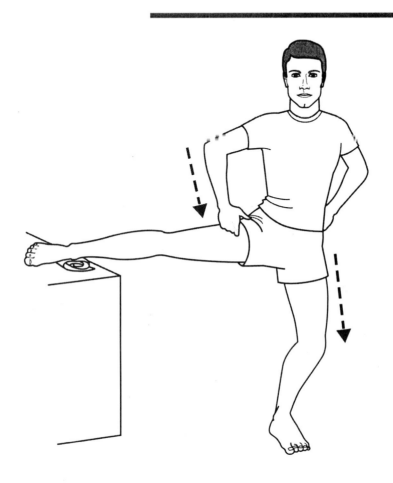

Figure 13-2

Suggestion(s) for Strengthening

Lie on side with involved hip down, top leg bent as shown in Figure 13-3. Raise bottom leg, hold briefly, then lower it. Ankle weights are optional.

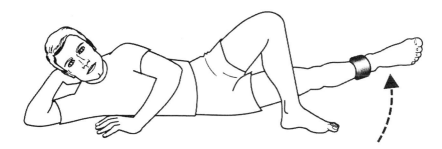

Figure 13-3

Lie on side with involved hip uppermost, lower leg slightly bent. Raise upper leg, hold briefly, then lower it. Ankle weights are optional. (See Figure 13-4.)

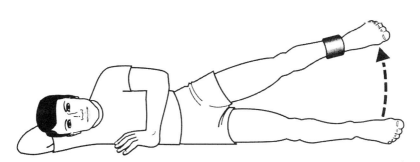

Figure 13-4

Notes and Contraindications

▶ Reminder: Failure to discover and correct for skeletal asymmetry is a major reason why many techniques and modalities fail to provide lasting, long-term musculoskeletal pain relief. If one side of the pelvis appears higher than the other but no skeletal asymmetries have been found, always recheck the arches of the feet, the leg length, and the height of the two halves of the pelvis. When taking the measurements, be sure that the feet are positioned as indicated in the instructions, that the arches are equal (or have been equalized), that the knees are straight, and that there is no lateral rotation at the pelvis.

Distortion: Anterior Pelvic Rotation

Chart Pattern

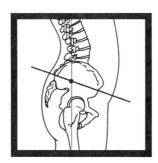

Goal

Stretch all muscles that tend to rotate or hold the pelvis anteriorly (forward); strengthen all muscles that tend to rotate or hold the pelvis posteriorly (backward). Note that only "pure crunches" should be done to strengthen the abdominals; while working to correct an anterior pelvic rotation, never do any abdominal strengthening exercise that brings the femurs (thigh bones) and the lumbar spine (low back) closer together or that involves tension between them, as in lifting or holding your legs and feet off the ground with your hips flexed. That kind of exercise necessarily uses and strengthens the hip flexors, precisely the opposite of what you're trying to achieve. Also, if your pelvis is rotated forward, do not strengthen your low back muscles; they are already short and tight as a result of having to pull your spine erect and hold it that way, so the last thing you want to do is make those lower back muscles any shorter and tighter than they already are. Stretch them instead. If the measurement is unclear, do a workout slightly unbalanced in the direction of correcting for anterior pelvic rotation.

What to Stretch

▶ Muscles that tilt the pelvis forward (hip flexors) (see Figure 13-5, Figure 13-6, and Figure 13-7), and muscles that pull the back upright (spinal extensors), especially in the low back (see Figure 13-8).

What to Strengthen

▶ Muscles that tilt the pelvis backward (abdominals) (see Figure 13-9), hip extensors (see Figure 13-10 and Figure 13-11).

Suggestion(s) for Stretching

Lie on a sturdy table, counter, or bench (the landing at the top of a flight of stairs also works well), with the edge under your sacrum as shown, not under your upper thighs. Pull one knee close to your chest, keeping your back as flat as possible, and let the other leg hang in a passive stretch. Alternate right and left legs. (See Figure 13-5.)

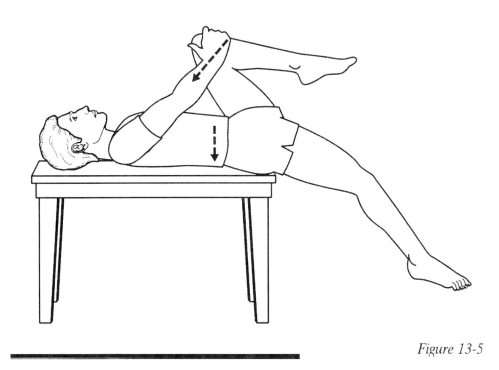

Figure 13-5

Lie prone in a push-up position, then raise your upper body *and pelvis* as shown in Figure 13-6, while *keeping your thighs on the floor.*

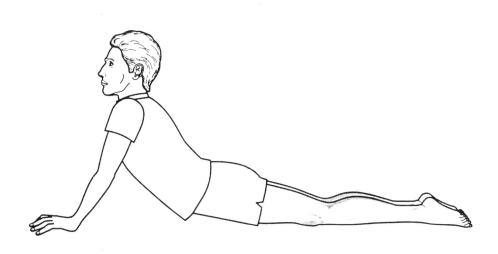

Figure 13-6

Lie along the edge of a low table, bench, bed, or couch with your off-table leg bent and the knee as close to your chest as possible. (See Figure 13-7.) Now reach back and pull your on-table foot toward your buttock. If you can't reach your foot, use a towel or belt wrapped around that ankle to pull with.

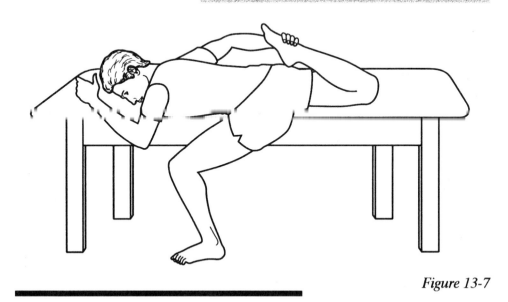

Figure 13-7

Sit with your legs in front of you and reach toward your toes. If desired, grasp legs and use arms to *gently* pull body forward to increase stretch. (See Figure 13-8.)

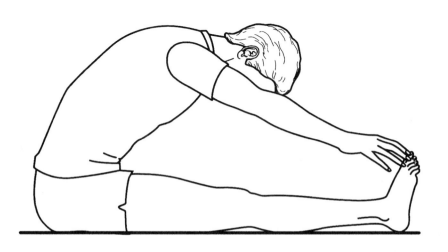

Figure 13-8

Suggestion(s) for Strengthening

As shown in Figure 13-9, lie on back with knees bent and feet resting on floor (if preferred, the backs of the heels can be rested on the seat of a chair). With hands behind head or across chest, lift upper body off floor, keeping low back flat on floor. Avoid bending neck forward with hands; instead, hold upper back and neck relatively straight, keeping eyes focused on a spot on the ceiling roughly over the feet. Never lift low back or feet off floor/chair, as this will engage the hip flexor muscles.

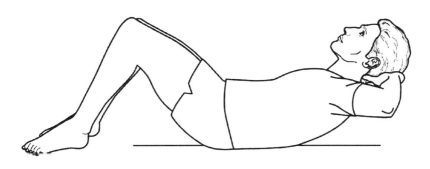

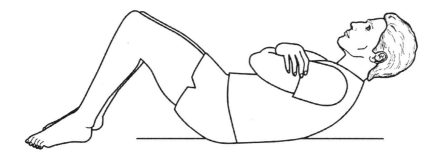

Figure 13-9

Lying prone, lift straight leg, hold briefly, then lower, alternating right and left legs. Ankle weights are optional. (See Figure 13-10.)

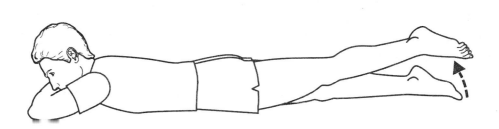

Figure 13-10

Lying prone, lift bent leg, hold briefly, then lower, alternating right and left legs. Ankle weights are optional. (See Figure 13-11.)

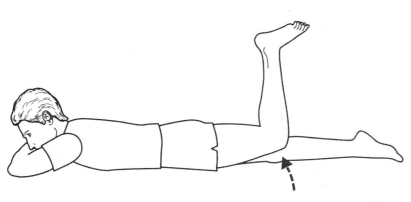

Figure 13-11

Notes and Contraindications

▶ When anterior pelvic rotation is found, always check carefully for anterior shoulder rotation and forward head posture, as they frequently accompany anterior pelvic rotation, especially when it is very pronounced.

▶ Anterior pelvic rotation is often a contributor to foot pain (especially in the forefoot) because the forward rotation of the pelvis moves the center of gravity forward, shifting more of the body weight to the balls of the feet and the toes.

Distortion: Posterior Pelvic Rotation

Chart Pattern

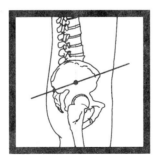

Goal

In this case, you want to do exactly the opposite of what you would do for anterior rotation: Stretch all muscles that tend to rotate or hold the pelvis posteriorly (backward); strengthen all muscles that tend to rotate or hold the pelvis anteriorly (forward). Consequently, because the hip flexors are weak, we want to strengthen them, so all those exercises that bring the femurs (thigh bones) and the lumbar spine (low back) together are now precisely what we want in order to strengthen the muscles that pull the pelvis forward and help restore the normal lumbar curve. Similarly, strengthening your lower back muscles so that they tighten and bow your lumbar spine forward into a normal curve is great, as long as you don't overdo it and eventually bow it too far forward. The advantage of using this method is that you can remeasure whenever you want, check to see how your body is changing, and adjust your workout accordingly. If the measurement is unclear, use a balanced workout, but with a slight emphasis toward correcting for an anteriorly rotated pelvis, as this is a much more common distortion than posterior pelvic rotation, especially if you spend a lot of time seated or in a hip-flexed position.

What to Stretch

▶ Muscles that tilt pelvis backward (hip extensors) (see Figure 13-12), abdominals (see Figure 13-13).

What to Strengthen

▶ Muscles that tilt pelvis forward (hip flexors) (see Figure 13-14) and muscles that pull the back upright (spinal extensors), especially in the low back (see Figure 13-15).

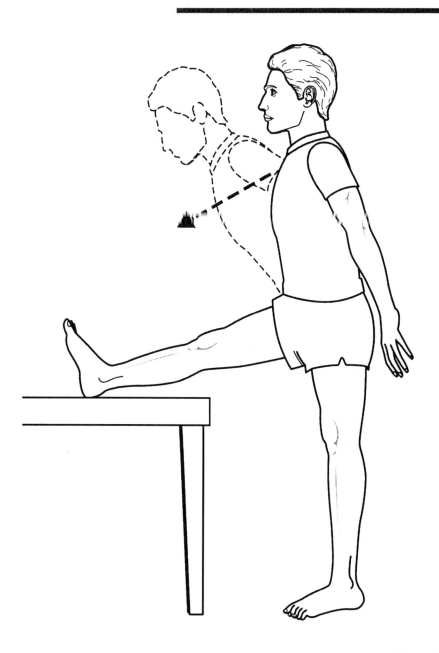

Figure 13-12

Suggestion(s) for Stretching

Place heel on elevated surface. Lean forward from the hip, keeping leg and back straight. (See Figure 13-12.)

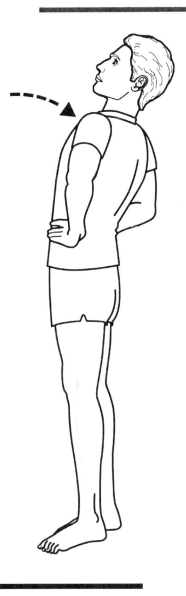

Figure 13-13

While standing with hands on hips (see Figure 13-13), slowly lean backward. Use caution with this stretch if you have disk problems in your lumbar spine.

Suggestion(s) for Strengthening

As shown in Figure 13-14 (see page 160), sit on an elevated surface, with feet not touching the ground. Slowly raise lower leg and straighten knee, then lower it. Ankle weights are optional. Another very effective way to strengthen the hip flexors, if there is no medical condition that precludes it, is to do a full or partial sit-up, similar to the abdominal crunch shown in Figure 13-9, except that in this case you *do* want to lift your low back off the floor and come up to, or at least toward, an upright sitting position.

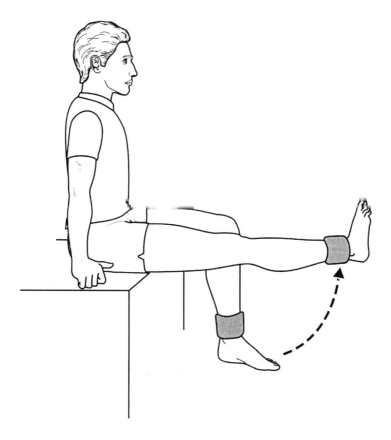

Figure 13-14

Lie on back and tighten back muscles to arch back upwards. Hold, then slowly lower back to floor. (See Figure 13-15.)

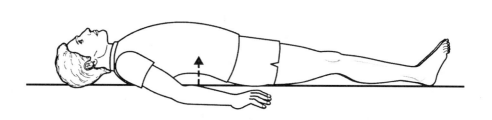

Figure 13-15

Notes and Contraindications

▶ When posterior pelvic rotation exists, always check for forward head posture, because the head tends to move anteriorly to counterbalance the posterior movement of the center of gravity in the pelvis.

Distortion: Lateral Pelvic Rotation

Chart Pattern

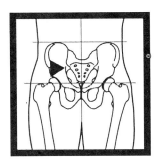

Goal

The pelvis should be balanced, with neither side more anterior than the other. If the measurement is unclear, assume the pelvis is not rotated and use a balanced workout.

What to Stretch

▶ Anterior side—Muscles that turn the leg outward (lateral hip rotators); see Figure 13-16.

▶ Posterior side—Muscles that turn the leg inward (medial hip rotators); see Figure 13-17.

What to Strengthen

▶ Anterior side—Muscles that turn the leg inward (medial hip rotators); see Figure 13-18.

▶ Posterior side—Muscles that turn the leg outward (lateral hip rotators); see Figure 13-19.

Suggestion(s) for Stretching

Lie face down as shown in Figure 13-16 with involved leg bent. Keeping pelvis and torso flat on floor, let bent leg rotate outward. Ankle weight is optional.

Stand with involved leg on support, as shown in Figure 13-17. Lean forward to increase stretch.

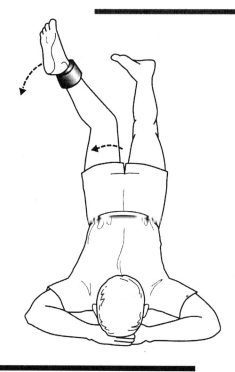

Figure 13-16

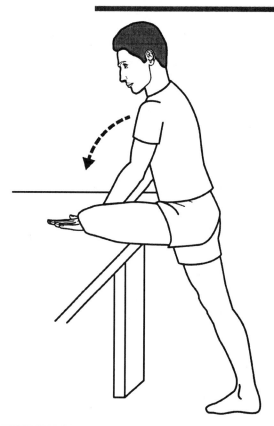

Figure 13-17

Suggestion(s) for Strengthening

Sit with anchored exercise tubing or resistance cable looped around ankle of involved leg, as shown in Figure 13-18. Keeping knees relatively close together, rotate ankle of involved leg outward. If necessary, stabilize knee position by clasping hands around active knee.

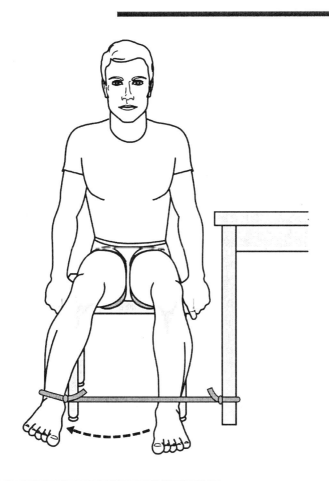

Figure 13-18

Sit with anchored exercise tubing or resistance cable looped around ankle of involved leg, as shown in Figure 13-19. Keeping knees relatively close together, rotate ankle of involved leg inward. If necessary, stabilize knee position by clasping hands around active knee.

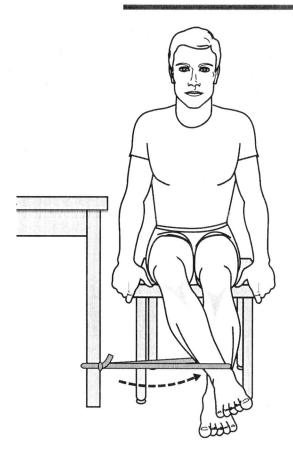

Figure 13-19

Notes and Contraindications

▶ If in doubt, always double check this measurement with leg lengths and arches corrected to be equal, if necessary, as unequal legs, unequal arches, or both can cause or exacerbate a lateral pelvic rotation.

Chapter 14

Stress Central:
Relieving the Neck and Shoulders

Alex had a powerfully built, athletic body, but the last three years of working 60 to 70 hours a week at his desk and computer had left him with intense, aching pain in his neck, shoulders, and upper back. I helped him understand that working for long periods with his hands in front of him had caused his chest muscles to tighten and remain shorter, thus pulling his shoulders and neck forward and causing the muscles at the back of his neck and shoulders to compensate by contracting constantly to keep his head erect and prevent it from falling forward. I suggested a home therapy program that included stretches for his tight chest, neck, and shoulder muscles, and he reported a couple of weeks later that the stretches really helped reduce his pain, even though he was still overworking his muscles by maintaining his intense work schedule.

Distortion: Lateral Shoulder Tilt

Chart Pattern

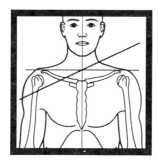

Goal

The shoulders should be level. A dropped shoulder can be caused by a fallen arch in the foot, a short leg, or a small hemipelvis, so those conditions should be ruled out or corrected first. When the sacral base (the top surface of the sacrum) has been leveled side to side, any remaining shoulder tilt is almost always due to muscular imbalance. If the measurement is unclear, consider the shoulders level and do a balanced workout.

What to Stretch

▸ High shoulder side—Muscles that elevate the shoulder (elevators of the scapula); see Figure 14-1.

▸ Low shoulder side—Muscles that pull the rib cage toward the pelvis (lateral trunk flexors); see Figure 14-2.

What to Strengthen

▸ High shoulder side—Muscles that pull the rib cage toward the pelvis (lateral trunk flexors); see Figure 14-3.

▸ Low shoulder side—Muscles that elevate the shoulder (elevators of the scapula); see Figure 14-4.

Suggestion(s) for Stretching

Sitting as shown in Figure 14-1a, with hand grasping seat of chair to stabilize involved shoulder, reach opposite hand over head and *gently* pull head away from shoulder. Also vary stretch by moving upper hand so it grasps head above and behind the ear, then pulling both toward opposite side and slightly forward. If seated on a couch or other long surface with no nearby edge to grasp, tuck hand under buttock as shown in Figure 14-1b and use arm strength to stabilize shoulder.

Standing as shown in Figure 14-2, raise arm and lean toward opposite side to stretch muscles on involved side.

Suggestion(s) for Strengthening

Standing with weight in opposite hand, slowly lift weight by leaning toward involved side, using only the muscles between the rib cage and pelvis on involved side. Hold briefly, then slowly lower weight and return to starting position. Keep pelvis still. (See Figure 14-3.)

Standing as shown in Figure 14-4, slowly raise involved shoulder to lift weight; hold briefly, then slowly lower weight. Be sure to keep head and torso still; don't rock to opposite side.

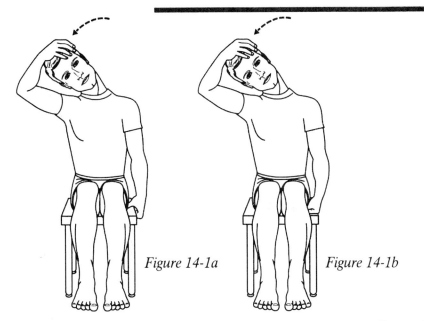

Figure 14-1a   Figure 14-1b

Figure 14-1

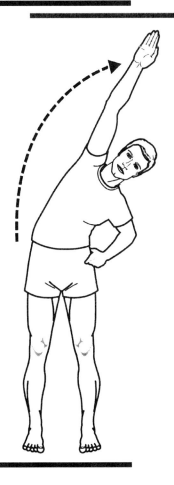

Figure 14-2

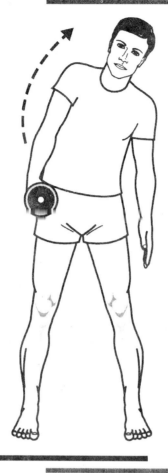

Figure 14-3

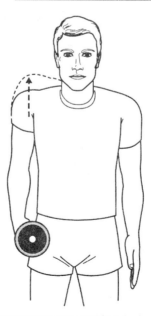

Figure 14-4

Notes and Contraindications

▶ Although it is not common, it is possible that an occasional individual may have a wedge-shaped vertebra, such that when looked at from the front or back, the vertebral body is not as tall (thick) on one side as it is on the other. This causes the vertebra above it to sit at an angle, resulting in a tilted spinal column above the wedge-shaped vertebra and consequent muscular compensation. A similar effect, also relatively uncommon, can be produced by a sacrum that is misaligned (that is, tilted to one side) within the pelvis itself. If you have any reason to suspect that either of these conditions might exist, consult a physician for a medical evaluation.

Distortion: Anterior Shoulder Rotation

Chart Pattern

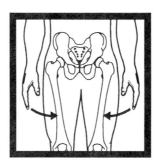

Goal

When viewed from the side, the center of the head of the humerus (the top of the upper arm bone) should be on the coronal plane, roughly in the middle of the body. However, it is extremely common to find one or both of the humeral heads pulled anteriorly and medially by tight chest muscles. If the measurement is unclear, do a workout slightly unbalanced in the direction of correcting for anterior shoulder rotation.

What to Stretch

▶ Muscles that move shoulder anteriorly (protractors of the scapula); see Figure 14-5.

What to Strengthen

▶ Muscles that move shoulder posteriorly (retractors of the scapula); see Figure 14-6, Figure 14-7, and Figure 14-8.

Suggestion(s) for Stretching

Stand with entire forearms (hands *and elbows*) resting on a doorframe or on adjoining walls, while facing into the corner. Keeping head erect, lean forward until a good stretch is felt across the chest. To lessen the stretch, move the feet closer to the doorway or corner; to increase it, move the feet farther out. If desired, one foot can be placed forward, toward the doorway or corner. Stretch can be varied, as shown, by keeping upper arms either a) angled upward, b) horizontal, or c) angled downward, thus emphasizing different parts of the chest muscles. (See Figure 14-5.)

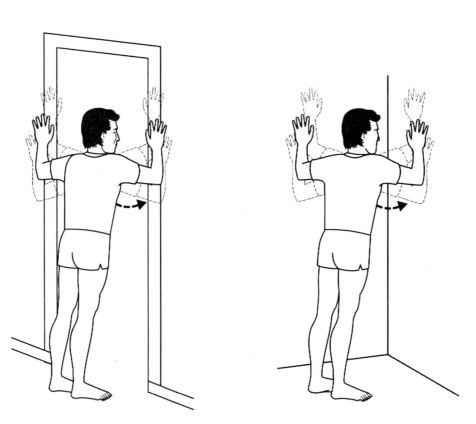

Figure 14-5

Suggestion(s) for Strengthening

Figure 14-6 shows four progressively more difficult variations of the same exercise. In (a), lying prone with hands at your sides, lift arms by pulling shoulder blades together; hold briefly, then slowly lower arms. Do not allow shoulders to move toward ears. In (b), hands are positioned alongside head, with elbows at right angles; lift arms as described in (a). In (c), arms are straight out to sides; lift arms as described in (a). In (d), arms are straight out to sides, with weights in hands; lift arms as described in (a).

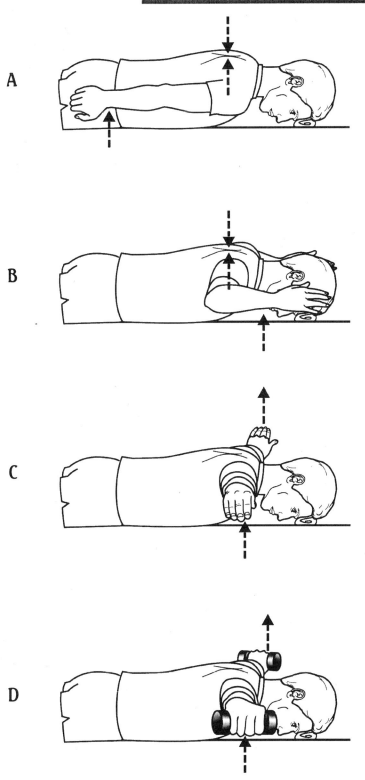

Figure 14-6

Keeping your shoulder blades pulled together and torso upright (see Figure 14-7), begin with arms straight out in front of you, grasping resistance tubing or handles of exercise machine. Pull against resistance, bringing arms in from fully extended position until upper arms are vertical by your side, as shown. Hold briefly, then slowly return to extended arm position.

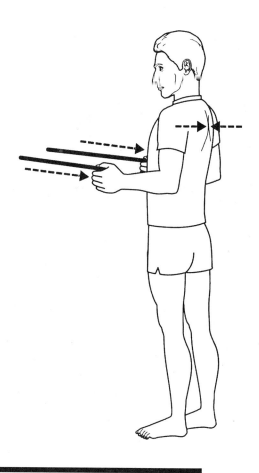

Figure 14-7

Keeping your torso upright (see Figure 14-8), begin with arms straight out in front of you, grasping resistance tubing or handles of exercise machine. Making sure to *keep elbows* straight, as shown in Figure 14-8, pull against resistance and bring shoulder blades together and slightly down. This is a small, precise movement of the shoulder blades; don't let your shoulders rise or your elbows bend in an effort to make it a larger movement than it needs to be. Hold briefly, then slowly return to start position.

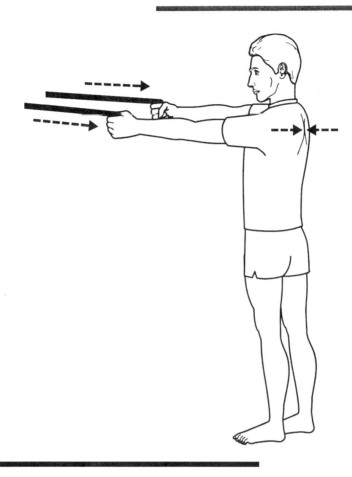

Figure 14-8

Notes and Contraindications

▶ When the shoulders are pulled anteriorly, the neck also tends to incline forward, causing you to look slightly downward, whether sitting or standing. As a result, the muscles in the back of the neck will be in constant contraction in order to tilt the head back and maintain a level gaze, so these muscles should be stretched also.

Distortion: Lateral Torso Rotation at Shoulders

Chart Pattern

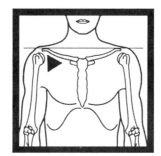

Goal

The shoulders at rest should be unrotated, with neither one more anterior than the other. If the measurement is unclear, consider the torso unrotated at the shoulders and do a balanced workout.

What to Stretch

▶ Muscles that turn the shoulders to one side (obliques); see Figure 14-9.

What to Strengthen

▶ Muscles that turn the shoulders to the opposite side (opposite obliques); see Figure 14-9.

Suggestion(s) for Stretching

Sitting with arms extended and wrapped around shoulder bar, as shown in Figure 14-9, rotate toward the *anterior (forward) shoulder* side *only*. Hold, then return to neutral position, facing forward.

Suggestion(s) for Strengthening

Same as "Suggestion(s) for Stretching." In addition, you can do a variation of the abdominal crunch shown in Figure 13-9. Lying on your back as shown with knees bent, turn your upper body as you lift it up so that the elbow on the side of the posterior shoulder moves toward the opposite knee. Do not lift your lower back or feet off the floor

Notes and Contraindications

▶ Remember that if the torso is forward at the shoulder on one side, the Righting Reflex will always produce a compensatory opposite rotation at the neck in order to enable the head to continue to face forward. Be sure to correct also for this lateral head rotation whenever a lateral torso rotation at the shoulder is found.

▶ If the shoulders have rotated to one side and the pelvis has either 1) remained unrotated; 2) rotated toward the opposite side; or 3) rotated to the same side as the shoulder, but not as much, it is necessary to stretch the oblique muscles that have produced that shoulder rotation—and strengthen the opposing obliques that rotate in the opposite direction—by doing the combination exercise and stretch shown in Figure 14-9, rotating the torso *toward* the *anterior shoulder* side. However, if the direction and degree of lateral rotation at the shoulders are the same as those at the pelvis, no correction of the oblique muscles is necessary, because the entire torso has rotated as a unit due to rotation at the pelvis. In this case, do a balanced workout of the obliques (as described above, but in both directions) and focus instead on doing the stretches and exercises to correct the lateral pelvic rotation, as well as the lateral head rotation that necessarily results from it.

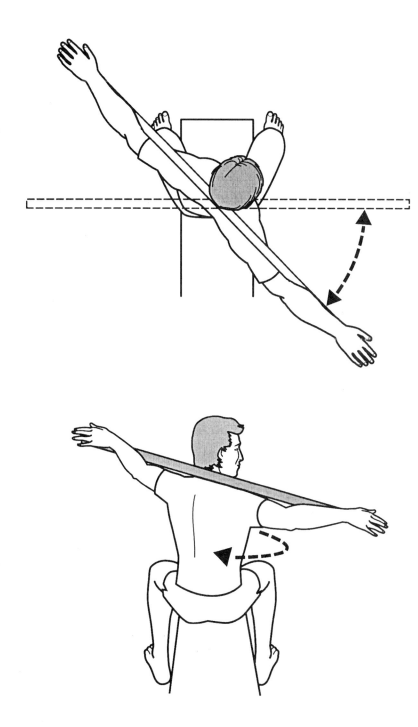

Figure 14-9

Distortion: Medial Rotation of Humerus

Chart Pattern

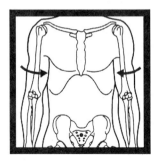

Goal

The arm should hang at the side of the body with the palm facing medially (toward the body). If the palm appears to be facing more posteriorly and the crease of the elbow is turned more medially than normal, the humerus is probably medially rotated. If the measurement is unclear, use a workout that is slightly unbalanced in the direction of correcting for medial humeral rotation.

What to Stretch

▶ Muscles that turn the upper arm inward (medial rotators of the humerus); Figure 14-10.

What to Strengthen

▶ Muscles that turn the upper arm outward (lateral rotators of the humerus); Figure 14-11.

Suggestion(s) for Stretching

Stand with elbows bent at right angles and hands on either side of doorframe, as shown in Figure 14-10. Lean entire body forward from ankles to create the stretch. If only one arm needs stretching, do the stretch as shown, but as you lean forward, turn your body toward the opposite arm to focus the stretch on the involved arm.

Suggestion(s) for Strengthening

Bend elbow of involved arm and grasp forearm with opposite hand. Keeping elbow of involved arm by your side, try to move forearm outward, resisting with opposite hand. (See Figure 14-11.)

Notes and Contraindications

▶ Judging medial rotation of the humerus by hand position alone can be misleading, as a posteriorly facing hand can also be caused by pronation of the forearm. To distinguish them, remember that medial humeral rotation will present an elbow crease and/or biceps that are facing more medially than normal, whereas pronation can occur with the elbow crease and biceps in a normal position, but with the hand still facing somewhat posteriorly. The two conditions can also occur together, requiring careful observation to distinguish the amount of distortion due to each.

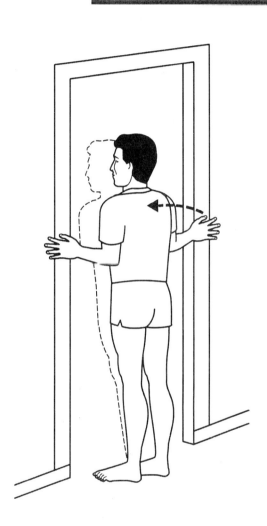

Figure 14-10

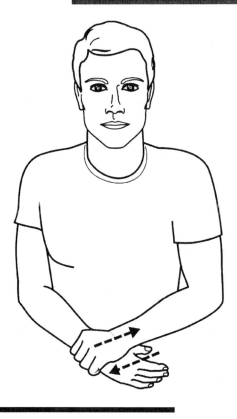

Figure 14-11

Distortion: Lateral Rotation of Humerus

Chart Pattern

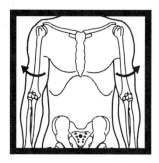

Goal

The arm should hang at the side of the body with the palm facing medially (toward the body). If the palm appears to be facing more anteriorly and the crease of the elbow is turned more laterally (outward) than normal, the humerus is probably laterally rotated. However, lateral rotation of the humerus is relatively uncommon, so if the measurement is unclear, use a balanced workout.

What to Stretch

▶   Muscles that turn the upper arm outward (lateral rotators of the humerus); see Figure 14-12.

What to Strengthen

▶   Muscles that turn the upper arm inward (medial rotators of the humerus); see Figure 14-13.

Suggestion(s) for Stretching

Stand as shown in Figure 14-12 with involved arm grasping towel behind back. Straighten other arm to increase stretch.

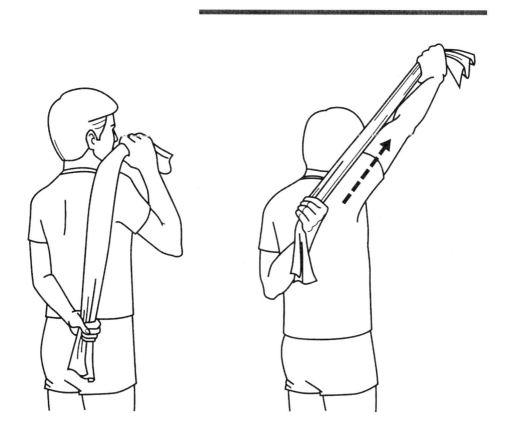

Figure 14-12

Suggestion(s) for Strengthening

Bend elbow of involved arm and grasp forearm with opposite hand. Keeping elbow of involved arm by your side, try to move forearm inward, resisting with opposite hand. (See Figure 14-13.)

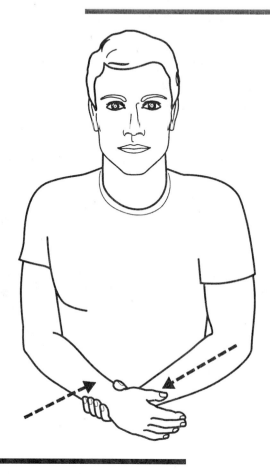

Figure 14-13

Notes and Contraindications

▶ Judging lateral rotation of the humerus by hand position alone can be misleading, as an anteriorly facing hand can also be caused by supination of the forearm. To distinguish them, remember that lateral humeral rotation will present an elbow crease and/or biceps that are facing more laterally (outward) than normal, whereas supination can occur with the elbow crease and biceps in a normal position, but with the hand still facing somewhat anteriorly. The two conditions can also occur together, requiring careful observation to distinguish the amount of distortion due to each.

Distortion: Forward Head Posture

Chart Pattern

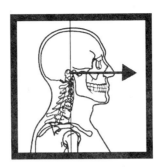

Goal

Viewed from the side, the external auditory meatus (the ear hole) should be on the coronal plane, directly over the center of the head of the humerus (essentially, the center of the shoulder). However, it is extremely common in our society to find a forward head posture. If the measurement is unclear, use a workout that is almost balanced but with a slight emphasis in the direction of correcting a forward head posture.

What to Stretch

▶ Muscles that move the head anteriorly and inferiorly (neck flexors) and muscles that tilt the head backward (posterior neck muscles); see Figure 14-14 and Figure 14-15.

What to Strengthen

▶ Muscles that move the head posteriorly and superiorly (anterior and posterior neck muscles); see Figure 14-16.

Suggestion(s) for Stretching

Move head backward and upward. Do not lift or drop chin; keep gaze level. If done properly, you should feel the stretch into the upper back and chest. (See Figure 14-14.)

Lying as shown in Figure 14-15, flatten neck by moving chin backward as head moves upward along surface. This can also be done while standing with your back against a wall and your feet slightly out from the wall.

Suggestion(s) for Strengthening

Lie on elevated surface with head hung over end (see Figure 14-16). Lift head so that neck is straight and level; hold briefly, then slowly lower to starting position.

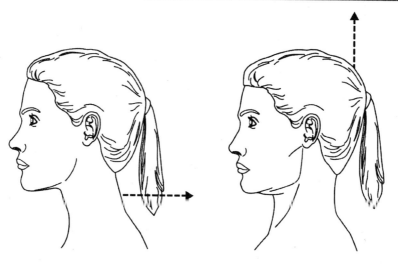

Figure 14-14

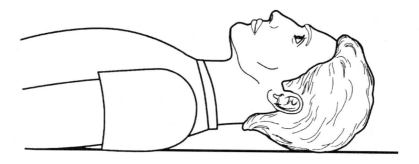

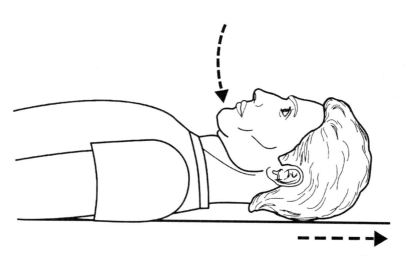

Figure 14-15

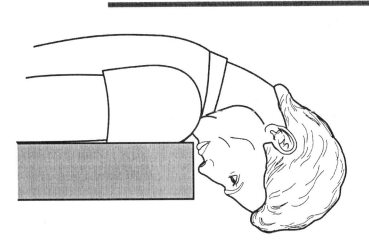

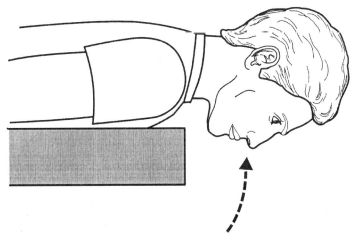

Figure 14-16

Notes and Contraindications

▶ Always perform all neck stretches and exercises gently. Never move the neck violently or suddenly, or with excessive force.

▶ If you have been diagnosed as having either a military neck or a reverse cervical curve, do *not* do the stretches and exercises suggested here unless they have been specifically approved by your physician.

▶ When the head is forward, the shoulders are also typically found to be pulled anteriorly. If this is the case, be sure to correct for anterior shoulder rotation as well.

Distortion: Lateral Head Rotation

Chart Pattern

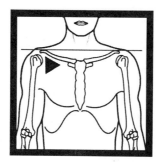

Goal

Whenever one shoulder is anterior with respect to the other, the upper part of the torso is turned toward the posterior shoulder, as a result of which the head rotates back toward the anterior shoulder so that you can maintain forward vision. If the shoulder measurement is unclear, use a balanced workout for the cervical rotators.

What to Stretch

▶ Muscles that rotate the head toward the anterior shoulder (cervical rotators); see Figure 14-17.

What to Strengthen

▶ Muscles that rotate the head toward the posterior shoulder (cervical rotators); see Figure 14-18.

Suggestion(s) for Stretching

Grasp head as shown in Figure 14-17 and rotate it gently toward the *posterior* shoulder.

Suggestion(s) for Strengthening

Rotate head toward *posterior* shoulder, resisting with hand. Hold briefly, then release. (See Figure 14-18.)

Notes and Contraindications

▶ Always perform all neck stretches and exercises gently. Never move the neck violently or suddenly, or with excessive force.

▶ When correcting for head counter-rotation that has occurred in response to the rotation of the shoulders, it is important to correct the shoulder rotation at the same time. Otherwise, the head rotation will recur in response to the continued rotation at the shoulders. Remember that, if the shoulders have rotated as a result of an equal rotation at the pelvis, the correction of the shoulder rotation must be made at the pelvis.

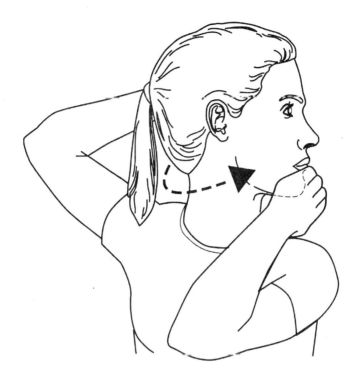

Figure 14-17

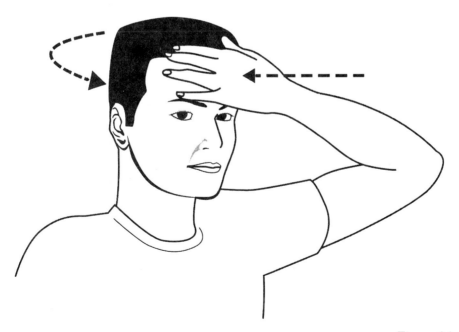

Figure 14-18

Chapter 15

High Intensity:
Calming the Arms, Hands, and Jaw

As were so many other talented computer programmers in 1999, Michelle was working incredible numbers of hours each week to try to prevent computer crashes on New Year's Day of 2000 due to the so-called Y2K bug. The endless hours at the keyboard left her with hands and forearms that throbbed and ached intensely, but she couldn't slow down or take time off because of the fast-approaching Y2K deadline. She felt trapped.

I showed Michelle how constant computer work required that certain arm and hand muscles remain in constant contraction, thus reducing blood flow to those muscles and bringing on pain, not only in those muscles, but in other pain-referral areas as well. I worked on her tight arm and hand muscles to get the relaxation started, then showed her simple exercises and stretches she could do at her desk to help keep them relaxed. As expected, she subsequently reported that whenever she did her exercises regularly, her pain decreased, but when she forgot or slacked off, her pain grew worse. She eagerly anticipated the day when the Y2K rush would be over so she could slow down, go back to working a normal workweek, and let her muscles fully heal.

Distortion: Elbow Flexion

Chart Pattern

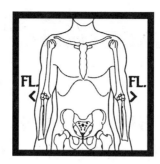

Goal

The arm should hang essentially straight at the side but is occasionally found flexed at rest, often as the result of exercising the elbow flexors more than the elbow extensors. If the measurement is unclear, use a balanced workout.

What to Stretch

▶ Muscles that bend the elbow (elbow flexors); see Figure 15-1.

What to Strengthen

▶ Muscles that straighten the elbow (elbow extensors); see Figure 15-2.

Suggestion(s) for Stretching

Lie on table or bed with pad on edge, which should be under upper arm. Let weight in hand straighten arm to produce stretch. (See Figure 15-1.)

Suggestion(s) for Strengthening

Lie as shown in Figure 15-2, supporting active arm with opposite hand. Starting with active elbow bent, raise weight until arm is vertical, hold briefly, then slowly lower to starting position.

Notes and Contraindications

▶ When doing the stretch shown here, care should be taken to select a weight that is not too heavy, as this could result in possible injury to the elbow joint. A light to moderate weight sufficient to produce a gentle stretch is best.

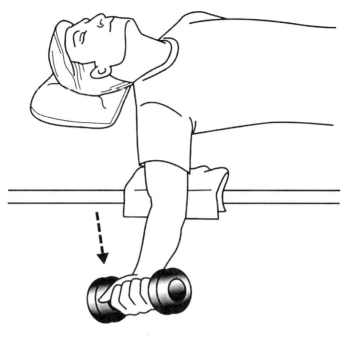

Figure 15-1

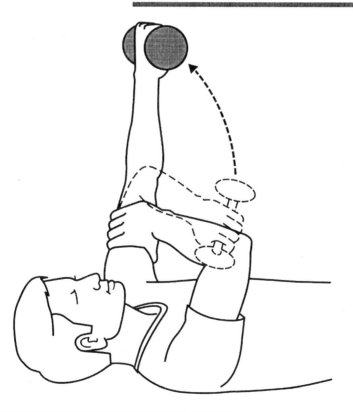

Figure 15-2

Distortion: Forearm Pronation

Chart Pattern

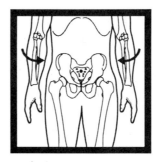

Goal

The arm should hang at the side with the palm facing medially. If the measurement is unclear, use a balanced workout, unless you spend extensive amounts of time with the forearms pronated (for example, typing, writing, playing the piano, and so on). In this case, use a workout that is unbalanced slightly in the direction of correcting for forearm pronation.

What to Stretch

▶ Muscles that turn the hand backward or palm down (forearm pronators); see Figure 15-3 and Figure 15-4.

What to Strengthen

▶ Muscles that turn the hand forward or palm up (forearm supinators); see Figure 15-3 and Figure 15-4.

Suggestion(s) for Stretching

These muscles are difficult to stretch effectively, and the complex instructions necessary to make sure that such stretching is done correctly would be out of place in this book. Because even the best attempt at stretching these muscles produces relatively little result, simply use the strengthening exercises shown in the following section for the opposing muscles, as that will naturally cause these muscles to relax.

Suggestion(s) for Strengthening

Sitting as shown in Figure 15-3, turn arm outward to lift weight on end of handle; hold briefly, then slowly let weight rotate inward and downward to the natural limit of the forearm. Be sure to stop outward rotation of handle well short of vertical position, as the last several degrees of weight travel are essentially horizontal and provide no significant resistance. If needed, a substitute source of resistance can be made by tying a weight (such as a soup can, or a bucket containing water or sand) to a piece of a broomstick. If a dumbbell is used, make sure that it has weight on only one end, not both.

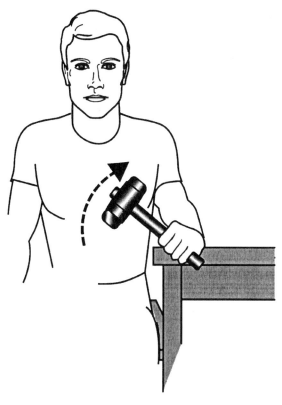

Figure 15-3

Grasp end of forearm near wrist, as shown in Figure 15-4. Try to turn forearm outward while resisting with grasping hand; hold briefly, then relax.

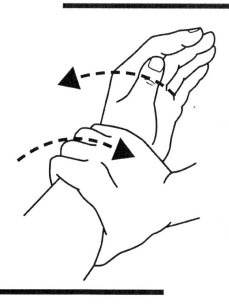

Figure 15-4

Notes and Contraindications

▶ Judging pronation of the forearm by hand position alone can be misleading, as a posteriorly facing hand can also be caused by medial rotation of the humerus. To distinguish them, remember that medial humeral rotation will present an elbow crease and/or biceps that are facing more medially (in toward the body) than normal, whereas pronation can occur with the elbow crease and biceps in a normal position, but with the hand still facing posteriorly. The two conditions can also occur together, requiring careful observation to distinguish the amount of distortion due to each.

Distortion: Forearm Supination

Chart Pattern

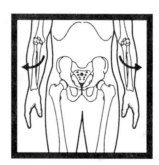

Goal

The arm should hang at the side with the palm facing medially. Compared to forearm pronation, forearm supination is relatively uncommon, so if the measurement is unclear, use a balanced workout.

What to Stretch

▶ Muscles that turn the hand forward or palm up (forearm supinators); see Figure 15-5 and Figure 15-6.

What to Strengthen

▶ Muscles that turn the hand backward or palm down (forearm pronators); see Figure 15-5 and Figure 15-6.

Suggestion(s) for Stretching

These muscles are difficult to stretch effectively, and the complex instructions necessary to make sure that such stretching is done correctly would be out of place in this book. Because even the best attempt at stretching these muscles produces relatively little result, simply use the strengthening exercises shown in the following section for the opposing muscles, as that will naturally cause these muscles to relax.

Suggestion(s) for Strengthening

Sitting as shown in Figure 15-5, turn arm inward to lift weight on end of handle; hold briefly, then slowly let weight rotate outward and downward to the natural limit of the forearm. Be sure to stop inward rotation of handle well short of vertical position, as the last several degrees of weight travel are essentially horizontal and provide no significant resistance. If needed, a substitute source of resistance can be made by tying a weight (such as a soup can, or a bucket containing water or sand) to a piece of a broomstick. If a dumbbell is used, make sure that it has weight on only one end, not both.

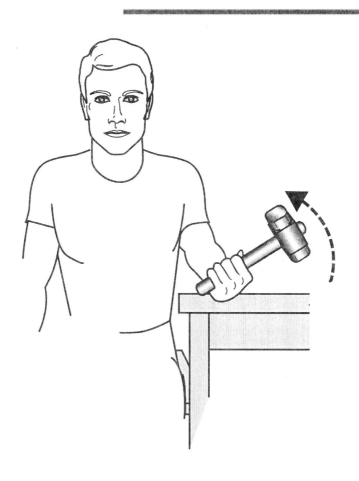

Figure 15-5

Grasp end of forearm near wrist, as shown in Figure 15-6. Try to turn forearm inward while resisting with grasping hand; hold briefly, then relax.

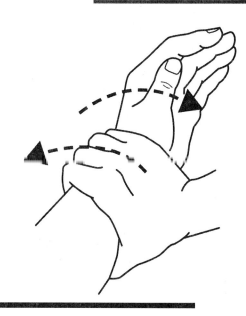

Figure 15-6

Notes and Contraindications

▶ Judging supination of the humerus by hand position alone can be misleading, as an anteriorly facing hand can also be caused by lateral rotation of the humerus. To distinguish them, remember that lateral humeral rotation will present an elbow crease and/or biceps that are facing more laterally (away from the body) than normal, whereas supination can occur with the elbow crease and biceps in a normal position, but with the hand still facing anteriorly. The two conditions can also occur together, requiring careful observation to distinguish the amount of distortion due to each.

Distortion: Finger Flexion

Chart Pattern

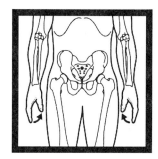

Goal

The arm should hang at the side with the fingers hanging nearly straight, having only a slight curve. If the measurement is unclear, use a balanced workout, unless you spend extensive amounts of time with the fingers curled (for example, typing, playing piano, gripping tools). In this case, use a workout that is unbalanced slightly in the direction of correcting for finger flexion.

What to Stretch

▶ Muscles that bend the fingers (finger flexors); see Figure 15-7.

What to Strengthen

▶ Muscles that straighten the fingers (finger extensors); see Figure 15-8.

Suggestion(s) for Stretching

With fingers spread far apart, pull fingers toward back of hand as far as possible. (See Figure 15-7.)

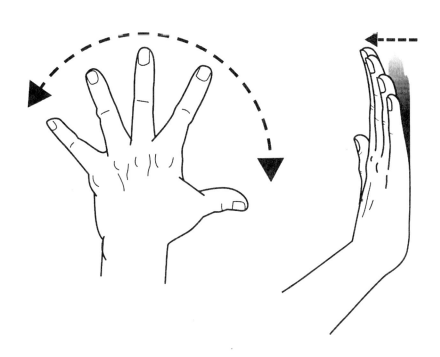

Figure 15-7

Suggestion(s) for Strengthening

With one or more thick rubber bands wrapped around fingers, spread fingers outward as shown; hold briefly, then slowly return to starting position. (See Figure 15-8.)

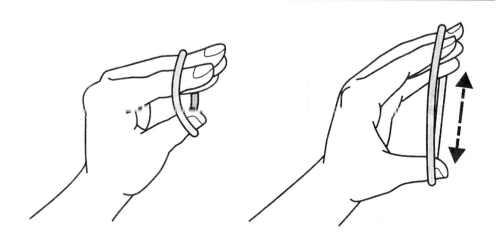

Figure 15-8

Distortion: Tight Jaw Muscles

Chart Pattern

Although tight jaw muscles are often found in conjunction with other postural distortions (for example, laterally tilted pelvis, anterior pelvic rotation, forward head posture), this condition cannot be confirmed by postural evaluation, so no chart pattern is available.

Goal

Tight jaw muscles are a common problem, often caused or exacerbated by postural distortion, and can result in TMJ (jaw joint) dysfunction, pain, clenching, and/or grinding of the teeth, so the goal is to stretch and relax the jaw muscles. Remember, though, that if there is an underlying postural distortion that is contributing to the muscle tension in the jaw, that underlying distortion must be corrected if the jaw muscle tension is to be resolved successfully on a long-term basis.

What to Stretch

▶ Muscles that close and clench jaws (elevators of the mandible); see Figure 15-9.

What to Strengthen

▶ Muscles that open jaws (depressors of the mandible).

Suggestion(s) for Stretching

Sit at table or desk as shown in Figure 15-9, bracing forehead with hand. With first two fingers and thumb of other hand, grasp lower jaw and gently traction it forward and down.

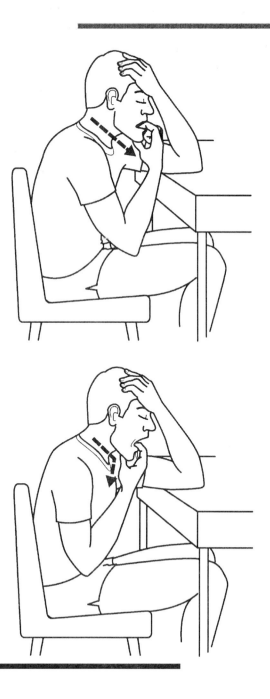

Figure 15-9

Suggestion(s) for Strengthening

Open the mouth as far as possible, as if yawning; hold briefly, then let jaws relax.

Notes and Contraindications

▶ Always perform all jaw stretches and exercises gently. Never use excessive force.

▶ If any TMJ dysfunctions or other jaw problems are present, or if you have any removable dentures or other dental appliances in the mouth, you should always obtain the approval of your supervising dentist, oral surgeon, or physician before doing any stretches or exercises involving the jaw.

▶ If the jaw muscles are extremely tight, it may be advisable to place a moist hot pack over the affected muscles in the area of the TMJ prior to attempting any jaw stretches or exercises.

Section IV

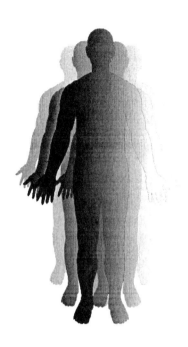

Staying Pain-Free

Chapter 16

If Your Pain Comes Back:
Creating Pain Relief for Life

As a housewife and mother of three children, Rachel stayed incredibly busy and had no time for the pain in the right side of her face and jaw, but years of doctor visits hadn't resolved the problem. I noted in her postural evaluation that her right shoulder was high and her left low, thus causing the muscles of her right shoulder to tighten to keep her head level, and the typical pain-referral pattern from those muscles matched her pain pattern exactly. I released the tight shoulder muscles and leveled her shoulders, then sent her home feeling much better. However, on each of her next two visits, when she came for other treatment, her right shoulder was slightly high again and her pain had come back, so each time I again released her muscles and leveled her shoulders.

At this point, I explained to Rachel that when a pain problem is resolved time after time but keeps coming back, there is a missing piece, a "perpetuating factor" that needs to be discovered and dealt with. I gave her the example of a receptionist, salesman, or attorney who spends all day with the phone held up to the ear by the shoulder muscles, thus retightening those muscles and recreating the pain. Her eyes grew wide. "That's me," she said. "Whenever I do my ironing, I call my best friend and talk as I work, and I'm holding the phone that way with my shoulder, sometimes for almost two hours at a time." I released her contracted muscles and leveled her shoulders yet again, then suggested that on the way home from my office she buy an inexpensive cordless phone with a headset and use it for all her calls, which she did. Because she no longer had to hold the phone to her ear with her shoulder muscles, her shoulders have remained level and her face and jaw pain has not returned.

Pain Relief for Life is not a "quick fix," a magic pill to be taken once and then forgotten. It involves becoming posturally conscious, making lifestyle changes, and developing a lifetime commitment to staying healthy, posturally balanced, and pain-free. Remember also that, although correcting postural distortion is an absolutely essential primary factor in getting rid of musculoskeletal pain, it is by no means the only factor. Although there have been dozens, if not hundreds, of books written about those other factors, it is important to review those other factors here briefly to help give you an appreciation of how they relate to the understanding you've gained from this book, as well as perhaps to give you ideas for further exploration.

One of the greatest benefits of the *Pain Relief for Life* system is that in addition to subjectively noticing your decreasing pain levels and your increased sense of well-being, you can easily monitor your progress objectively simply by doing another postural evaluation. Some distortions, such as a shoulder tilt or forearm pronation, can be monitored just by looking in the mirror; others can be checked by getting together with your partner and reevaluating each other. Although of course you can do a postural evaluation as often as you like, the program needs time to work, so it's normally not worthwhile to do a complete reevaluation more often than about every two or three months, though you may want to do a quick check on one or two particular distortions more frequently. The important thing is that it's your body and your pain, so it's up to you; you're in charge now. Evaluate as often as you feel is needed, then adjust your pain relief program as discussed in Chapter 10 under "Principles of Postural Pain Relief."

If your postural distortions are improving and your pain is decreasing, that's great, but what if they aren't? In that case, recheck your measurements, then make sure that you've marked them correctly on your chart and that you're doing the right corrections for the distortions you found. (If you're in doubt, refer to the Chart Pattern icons in Section III; they're there to help you make sure that you're on the right track.)

What if the pain comes back? Suppose you've measured correctly, created and followed your program for a while, and resolved your pain, yet all of a sudden it starts to return. When this happens, you need to look for a "perpetuating factor," a hitherto unrecognized source of pain, often from postural distortion. Typically this is something you do regularly or frequently in the course of your daily activities, and usually without thinking about its impact on your posture and your pain. Although the possibilities here are almost endless, a quick list of examples (some from cases mentioned earlier) will help to give you an idea of the kinds of things to look for:

▸ Leaning to one side while driving, using the computer, or watching TV.

▸ Using a mouse with your "mouse arm" held way out to the side or far in front of you.

▸ While using a computer, tilting your head up or down because of using the wrong glasses or to avoid screen glare.

▸ Turning your head to use a computer monitor located to the right or left of your keyboard

▸ Holding the telephone to your ear with your shoulder.

▸ Habitual or frequently assumed postures, such as crouching or bending over, whether in work or in sports (such as skiing, bicycle racing, speed skating, or playing pool).

▸ Always carrying heavy weights, such as purses or luggage, in one hand or over one shoulder.

▸ Prolonged hip flexion for any reason, including sitting at work, driving or flying, riding horseback, playing the piano, and so forth.

▸ Prolonged forward head posture, such as generally occurs when sitting or standing in a slumped posture, working over a desk, driving or flying, leaning over students or patients, reading, doing knitting or other handicrafts, and so on.

▸ Frequently moving or twisting the body to one side more than the other, as in swinging a golf club or baseball bat, or in some repetitive motion at work.

You can also look for other non-postural perpetuating factors, such as:

▸ Using a foam pillow, the springiness of which can aggravate neck and shoulder pain; try a feather pillow instead.

▸ Having short upper arms. When standing, your upper arm should reach to the iliac crest, the top of your pelvis; if it's shorter, it can cause shoulder and neck strain when sitting. Raise or build up the arms of your chairs.

▸ Wearing constricting clothing that puts pressure on muscles, such as thin bra straps across the shoulder muscles or tight collars on neck muscles.

▸ Using desks, chairs, or other furniture not properly sized for you, causing muscular strain as your body tries to adapt.

The key here is to use your new knowledge to examine even the most mundane activities in your life and to see if any of them could be contributing to your postural distortion and creating your pain. Because it's not possible to focus on your posture at every instant of your life, it's often helpful to have a "nagging buddy," someone (perhaps a spouse or coworker) to keep an eye on you and remind you (nicely!) if you tend to slump, tilt, twist, sit, or stand in some way that you're not aware of. Not only can this provide you with information that you might otherwise miss, it might also encourage your "nagging buddy" to become more posturally aware and start making his or her own changes.

The effect of correcting for a perpetuating factor can sometimes be striking. Some years back, I was teaching a seminar in a city in the Midwest and was asked by a local therapist if I would see a client of hers, a young woman in her late 20s who never seemed to remain out of pain. The therapist was excellent and had worked frequently on this woman (I'll call her Samantha) over the preceding two years, and although Samantha had gotten better each time she always seemed to regress and wind up in pain again. In the course of a thorough postural evaluation, I noted that Samantha had one hemipelvis that appeared to be about 3/16-inch smaller than the other in its vertical dimension. I had her sit on a nearby table, then fashioned a makeshift 3/16-inch support out of my teaching manual that was lying nearby and stuck it under her smaller hemipelvis in order to make the pelvis level.

The result was instantaneous. No sooner had she settled down onto the support than tears welled up in her eyes; this was the first time in her life, she told me, that she had been able to sit without pain. She was overjoyed, and when I asked her to raise her buttock so that I could have my manual back, she laughingly refused, saying that it felt so good that she was never going to give it back. I also tested her for the appropriate correction needed in the standing position, with similar results. Since then she has been careful to support herself appropriately whenever she is standing or sitting, and the relief of her pain has been nothing short of remarkable.

Whatever the underlying cause of any pain, one of the primary triggers that can cause that pain to suddenly appear or increase is stress. I've seen it time and again, both in my practice and in my own life: Whenever you have any chronic condition that flares up periodically—be it muscle pain, headaches, indigestion, stomach cramps, colds, flu, allergies, skin rashes, or whatever—always take a moment to check your stress level whenever that condition suddenly reappears or worsens significantly, especially if it's for no other known reason. If you're both thorough and honest in your self-evaluation, chances are you'll find that your stress meter is reading a bit on the high side. Although this is not a book on stress reduction (there are plenty of those available), it is important to emphasize here that even the best pain-reduction program will have only limited success if it is fighting an uphill battle against an overwhelming load of stress. Doing the corrective stretches and exercises in this book will actually go a long way toward reducing the physical component of your overall stress load, but if you're highly stressed it's crucial that you also address the other components of your stress if you want to achieve long-term pain relief.

In order to keep our stress levels at a minimum, it is vital that we keep ourselves in good health—physical, emotional, mental, and spiritual. If any of these begin to degrade, our stress levels can rise and our pain conditions can begin to manifest or get worse. Many years ago, a woman in her 40s came to me for help with crippling headaches and neck and shoulder pain that she'd had for years. It was only after she felt secure in our therapeutic relationship that she finally told me that she had been raped when she was in her early teens. Her posture, both sitting and standing, reflected her emotions exactly. Her upper body was curled forward, with her shoulders likewise pulled forward as if to come around and protect her heart from further wounding, and the only parts of the fetal position that were missing were the hands and knees drawn up to the chest. Although I was able to help her somewhat in reducing her physical pain, I explained to her that no pain relief we had achieved would ever be lasting until she got help with the emotional and mental issues that so dominated her life that they had become manifest in her posture. Fortunately, she did seek help in those other areas and her pain ultimately decreased significantly.

Additionally, it's important not to forget the basics: good nutrition and hydration, regular exercise, and plenty of relaxation and sleep. After all, it's hardly logical to expect that the muscles in a body stressed by a poor diet, improper hydration, lack of exercise, and insufficient sleep will recover and be as pain-free as those in a body that receives proper care. The good news, though, is that all of this is totally under your—and only your—control (if in doubt on this, please reread "Philosophy 101" in the Introduction).

Tips, Tricks, and Suggestions for Staying Pain-Free

In addition to using your personal pain-relief program, here are a few ideas to help you reduce or eliminate pain.

Tennis Balls

For quick relief of painful areas anywhere in the hard to reach back or hip areas, a tennis ball does wonders. Either place it on the floor and lie on it to put pressure on the painful area, or else stand with your back next to a wall, take a wide stance for good balance, bend your knees slightly, then place the tennis ball behind your back, using your legs to create pressure against the ball, and roll up, down, and sideways on the wall to work the sore area. When you buy a can of three tennis balls, it's a good idea to keep one at home, one at the office, and the third in your suitcase at all times so that relief is never far away, even when you're traveling.

Driving

When driving, always sit upright and be sure that your mirrors are positioned so that you have to sit upright in order to use them properly, as this can help to prevent slumping. Always be sure to use a good lumbar support; although many cars come equipped with lumbar supports now, many of those supports are either inadequate or poorly positioned, especially if you are significantly shorter or taller than average. If in doubt, fold an old towel in half along its length so that it's about as wide as you are, roll it up tightly from one end and secure it with some string or duct tape, then put it behind the small of your back, as follows. Being sure to keep your sacrum against the back of the seat, lean forward and slip the rolled towel in just above your belt line, then lean back and notice how this position causes your shoulders and head to sit back instead of slumping forward and causing neck, back, and head pain. If this improves the way you feel when you drive, adjust the position and/or thickness of the lumbar roll until it feels just right. This can really make a huge difference in your comfort level, especially on long trips. It's also a good idea to stop at least once an hour and take a couple of minutes to stretch, especially your hip flexors, which you can do somewhat by simply leaning backward (see Figure 13-13). Also, it's a good idea to do some neck stretches (see Figure 14-1) while you're at it; not only will you feel better, but you'll also be more alert.

Poor arm position while driving is another frequent source of pain. Holding the top of the wheel with one arm locked straight tends to raise that shoulder, causing your neck and shoulder muscles to contract to hold your head upright, while holding the wheel with both arms locked straight causes tension in both shoulders and the neck. Instead, try driving with "sandbag arms"—that is, letting your arms sag while holding the wheel as if they were filled with sand. If your car is designed so that you can use some part of the car as an armrest for one or both elbows while still holding the wheel properly, by all means do so in order to give your shoulders a rest.

By the way, when buying a car, although a fancy paint job and a great stereo system may be nice, it's infinitely more important to test drive the car to see how it fits you posturally. Take time to see whether the seat supports you properly or makes you slump, whether your arms can rest naturally when you hold the wheel or cause strain in your shoulders, and so on. Remember: You're going to be driving this vehicle for thousands and thousands of miles; why buy a vehicle that will only cause you pain? If you tell the car dealer that you won't buy that car because it's poorly designed, who knows, maybe the message will ultimately filter back to the car designers and they'll start making cars that are posturally correct and comfortable. For example, some of us are old enough to remember when some cars had not only tilt steering wheels but telescoping steering columns, one of the best postural features ever designed into a car, as they allowed the driver to position the seat as far back as necessary for appropriate leg room, then move the steering wheel closer or farther away to create ideal arm and shoulder comfort, thus allowing the car to be customized to fit each driver. Perhaps, if enough of us demand posturally correct cars, we can get all the car manufacturers to offer such features again.

Flying

I am convinced that most airline seats were originally designed as instruments of torture. Instead of giving support in the lumbar area, many of them are actually concave, thus allowing your low back to bulge posteriorly and causing your shoulders and head to jut forward. Nor is this postural cruelty limited to the seats in the coach section: A number of the so-called "first-class" seats, though wider and roomier, have a built-in pillow pad behind the head that forces the head into a forward head posture for the duration of the flight. Much as when driving, the only solution is to support your low back by putting a pillow, a rolled-up blanket, or a folded sweater behind your lumbar spine, just above the belt line, adjusting as necessary until your shoulders and head can sit back naturally and relax. Also, just as when driving, it's good to get up and stretch at least once an hour, especially on long flights.

Skyhook Walking

Many people unknowingly contribute to their postural distortion and pain by slumping or slouching as they trudge along. If I've just described you, try what I call "Skyhook Walking" instead. Imagine that there's a big skyhook that follows you everywhere, lifting you up by a cable attached to the top of your head, so that your shoulders hang from your torso like a suit jacket hanging on a clothes hanger. Standing on your toes, feel the skyhook letting your body down just enough so that your heels lightly touch the ground; then, letting the skyhook continue to hold you erect, start walking "over" the ground, rather than trudging "on" it. You should feel yourself walking with a smooth stride, an erect carriage, and a slight tension in the upper back as your muscles hold you upright and keep you from slumping. If you consistently walk with this new upright posture, not only will you help eliminate postural distortion and pain, you'll also look better and feel better psychologically, because this posture brings your chest out, your shoulders back, and helps you to "face life squarely." Try it for a while and see. Another way to help achieve the same effect is to walk with a five-pound sandbag on your head, though I suspect you may find Skyhook Walking a better choice when you're out in public!

Also, when walking, note whether your arms swing exactly parallel to your line of motion or instead swing somewhat diagonally across in front of you. The latter is a sign that your shoulders are anteriorly rotated, so try to keep your shoulders back by pulling your shoulder blades together until your arm swing on both sides is parallel to your line of motion. Periodically check your arm swing again, or have a companion keep an eye on it, until it becomes an ingrained habit to walk with your shoulders back.

Desk and Computer Work

Because sitting at a desk for hours on end is a surefire recipe for posturally induced pain, here are a few tips that can help to make you more comfortable:

- Whenever you have to sit for prolonged periods of time, set a timer for 30 minutes and place it across the room so that when it rings or beeps you have to actually get up from your seat to shut it off. Once you're up, take at least 30 to 60 seconds to stretch (the Doorway/Corner Stretch shown in Figure 14-5 is one great choice), then reset the timer before you sit down again. This will help keep you feeling fresher and less contorted.

- Given a choice, always use a desktop computer in preference to a laptop, unless the laptop is in a docking station with a separate, properly positioned monitor and keyboard. Although standalone laptops are sometimes a necessary evil, their inherent design forces you to tilt your head forward and down to look at the screen, resulting in neck and shoulder pain, and frequently headaches as well.

- Keep your monitor directly in front of you, with the center of the screen no more than about two inches below your horizontal line of sight. Keep the screen glare-free, either by correcting the room lighting or using a glare-reducing screen cover.

- Make sure your eyeglasses are correct for computer use and don't cause you to tilt your head up or down in the slightest in order to be able to see the screen properly. If in doubt, have your glasses checked or get special glasses made for computer use.

- Position your keyboard at such a height and such a distance from you that your upper arms can rest naturally at your sides and your forearms can be essentially horizontal. The same goes for your mouse; locate your mouse pad so that your "mouse upper arm" can rest next to your body as much as possible, reaching neither forward nor to the side, and your "mouse forearm" is horizontal.

> ▶ Because upper arm lengths vary, chair armrests with a fixed height won't fit everybody. Whenever possible, use a chair with adjustable arm rests and keep the arms set so that when you are sitting naturally upright you neither have to slump because the arm rests are too low, nor find your shoulders forced upward because the arm rests are too high. If your upper arms are too short or the chair armrests are too low, add padding on top of the chair arms to build them up.

Fingers

If you do a lot of typing, gripping of tools, or other intense hand work, your fingers may start to curl, rather than hanging straight, so it's helpful to counterbalance that overuse by doing corrective finger spreads (see Figure 15-7) and rubber band spreads (see Figure 15-8) during otherwise unproductive time, such as while you're talking on the phone, watching TV, or sitting in your car at a traffic light.

Shoes

As Dr. Victor Barker so elegantly shows in his superb book, *Posture Makes Perfect,* the elevation of the heels of shoes is a fad that caught on about 400 years ago and unfortunately has been wreaking postural havoc and causing untold pain ever since. There is no design flaw in the human body that requires the heel of the foot to be elevated in order to function properly. If someone asks, well, what about having to cushion the heel in sports, you need look no farther than those marvelous runners from some African countries who triumph barefoot in international long distance running competitions. All that elevating the heel of a shoe does is to throw the body out of postural alignment by tilting the body forward, thus requiring the muscles in the back of the body to remain in constant contraction to keep the torso upright and contorting the weight-bearing joints, and the higher the heel, the greater the postural distortion and pain. Simply put, the flatter a shoe is, the better it is from a postural/pain relief point of view; just cover and protect the feet, don't tilt them.

The Spinal Roll and Sacral Pad

One gentle way to stretch tight chest muscles is to place a towel on the floor, roll it up from its long side, creating a long, thick, tightly-rolled pad no more than about two to three inches in diameter, then lie down on the roll so that it lies under and supports your head and spine, preferably all the way to your sacrum. The idea is for the roll to lift your head and spine while letting gravity pull your shoulders down on either side of the roll, so be sure that the roll lifts your torso high enough that your shoulders are off the ground and that it fits between your shoulder blades so that it isn't preventing them from being pulled down by gravity. This spinal roll can easily be used while watching TV or listening to music.

A similar technique can be used to ease tight sacroiliac joints, the joints on either side of your sacrum where the upper part of the two halves of the pelvis are heavily bound to the sacrum by strong ligaments. To do this, you can use a rolled or folded washcloth or tiny towel, and the idea here is to lift the sacrum high enough that the two halves of the pelvis are lifted off the ground and the ligaments around the sacroiliac joints can be gently stretched as gravity, aided by the weight of the upper legs, pulls the two halves of the pelvis down on either side of the sacral pad you've created. In this case, however, you need to make sure that the sacral pad is narrow enough that it only lifts the sacrum and isn't under the mating edges of the two halves of the pelvis. Although the amount of movement possible in these sacroiliac joints is normally very tiny, even a slight reduction of pressure in the joint can sometimes bring noticeable relief.

To do this, you first have to locate the bony lump on either side of the top of the sacrum, a structure called the posterior superior iliac spine, or PSIS for short. Sit on the front edge of a chair and place your hands on your sacrum with the fingertips meeting at your coccyx or tailbone, just above the seat of the chair. Your sacrum sits like an upside-down arrowhead with its point just above the coccyx, so, keeping your fingertips flat, feel for the edges of the sacrum and work your way upward and outward along the edges until you feel a marble-sized lump of bone just inside either edge of the sacrum, just below the belt line. As you lie on your sacral pad, it should be narrow enough to fit between, but not under, these two bony landmarks. If you want to increase the effect of gravity somewhat, try lifting your knees toward your chest so that the entire weight of your legs is over your pelvis as you lie on the pad.

Standing

One way to help reduce back pain if you have to stand in one place for a long time is to put one foot up on an elevated footrest of some kind. That brass rail on the floor around the bar that you see in pictures of old saloons wasn't there because the owners had extra money in the decorating budget; it was there because when patrons could put one foot up on the rail, they'd be more comfortable standing at the bar and would stay longer and drink more. If you have to stand at a copy machine for a long time, try putting one foot up on a box of copier paper or an inverted wastebasket. If you're washing a lot of dishes in the sink, you can open the cabinet under the sink and put one foot up on the ledge inside.

Sleeping

From a postural standpoint, sleeping on your back is ideal if you have no medical problems that make that inadvisable. If doing so causes you low back discomfort, try sleeping with a pillow under your knees. Sleeping on your side is second best, as long as your mattress and pillow keep your spine aligned horizontally, although it does push your bottom shoulder forward and allow your top shoulder to fall forward with gravity, so your shoulders spend the night in an anteriorly rotated position, thus allowing your chest muscles to adaptively shorten. (Stretch them when you get up, as in Figure 14-5.) If side sleeping causes you hip pain in your uppermost hip, try sleeping with a pillow between your knees. Sleeping on your stomach is tough on your low back and devastating to the neck, as the prone position forces you to sleep with your head turned to one side in order to be able to breathe. Lying in that position all night will wreak havoc on your neck and back muscles; avoid stomach sleeping if at all possible. Also, if you have protracted neck and shoulder pain, avoid using a foam pillow, as the springiness of the foam can irritate trigger points in the neck and shoulder muscles; try a feather pillow instead, folding it double if you need greater thickness in order to keep your cervical spine aligned while sleeping on your side.

Chapter 17

A World Without Pain:
Spreading the Word and Helping Others

Christy had suffered for years from frequent abdominal pain that usually radiated into her low back. After more doctor visits than she could remember and numerous medical tests, all of which were negative, she came to my office at the urging of a friend. A quick glance at her hip-flexed posture led me to suspect trigger points in her shortened hip flexor muscles. When I pointed to a chart on the wall that showed the characteristic pain referral pattern of these muscles, she exclaimed, "That's it; that's exactly where my pain is!"

I explained to Christy that her tight hip flexors were due primarily to all the sitting she had to do for her job, but were made worse by the fact that some of the exercises in her workout program at the gym were in fact causing her hip flexors to tighten even further. I assured her that I could release a lot of the tightness in her hip flexors with neuromuscular therapy, but that she could take charge of her own pain relief by simply changing her workout to only stretch her contracted hip flexors while counterbalancing all her sitting by strengthening the opposing muscles, her hip extensors. As I worked on her, she felt her contracted muscles slowly but surely relax and noticed the pain decreasing in her abdomen and low back. All of a sudden, I noticed tears in her eyes, and her voice shook with frustration and anger as she asked the question I'd heard so many times: "Why hasn't anybody told me this before? This all makes such perfect sense; it's so logical and straightforward. When I think of all the time and money I've wasted on useless treatments…all those years I spent in pain and didn't have to…." Her voice trailed off and her tears flowed in silence.

Postural distortion isn't the cause of all pain, nor is the correction of postural distortion a "magic bullet" that will solve every pain problem; however, the lack of attention to postural distortion has resulted in an absolute epidemic of unnecessary pain, misery, and expense. Every one of you can help to make a major step forward in the improvement of healthcare in this country and around the world. And, please, this does **not** take a government program to achieve; governments tend to make almost everything they do hopelessly inefficient and unnecessarily expensive—and besides, this is all about personal responsibility, remember? (If you don't remember, please reread the part of the Introduction entitled "Philosophy 101.") All it takes is individuals demanding to be posturally measured and evaluated in order to get things to start changing. Get active in your own pain-relief program and encourage others to do likewise. If we start now, not only can we significantly reduce the cost of healthcare, but in a single generation we could sharply reduce the scourge of musculoskeletal pain caused by skeletal asymmetry and poor posture.

Although modern medicine is often capable of making very difficult diagnoses and achieving stunning results in treatment, its approach has become very biochemical, and simple structural analysis is all too often left out of the medical evaluation. This is unfortunate, as my clinical experience has convinced me that untreated postural distortion is responsible for much of the musculoskeletal pain in the world today, and in particular that uncorrected skeletal asymmetries constitute a major root cause of the veritable epidemic of back, hip, neck, and head pain currently afflicting our modern society. The solution, thankfully, is both easy and inexpensive to implement: universal screening for postural distortion and skeletal asymmetries.

Although this may sound like a monumental undertaking, it needn't be. If every physician or clinic took one minute—60 seconds—with each new patient to screen for significant skeletal asymmetries, that step alone would catch a huge percentage of those cases early on. If each physician or clinic had someone on staff trained to do a full postural evaluation (similar to the one outlined in this book, only in greater detail) and offer appropriate advice on corrective stretching and exercise, it could help millions of people worldwide to reduce or eliminate their own pain without drugs or surgery, as well as save many of them from the ill effects that can be caused by the prolonged pressure on the organs caused by postural distortion.

This approach is "low tech," is inexpensive, and will help greatly to reduce medical costs, both for individuals and for society as a whole, thus helping to keep health insurance rates lower as well. These benefits are especially important in poorer countries where the availability of high-tech medicine is limited and resources are scarce, because this approach would identify and resolve the posturally induced cases and thereby allow the overworked physicians in such countries to focus their limited time and resources on the more serious cases.

Although the evaluation of postural distortion and skeletal asymmetries is important for all people, there are certain groups who would especially benefit if such evaluation were to become universal. Some examples follow.

A Word to Athletic Coaches and Team Owners

Every athlete—amateur, Olympic, or professional—should be on a level structural foundation and posturally balanced if top performance is to be achieved. Too many careers have been needlessly hampered or cut short by back pain or muscle injuries that could have been prevented if the skeletal foundation and posture had been optimized. I've tested the muscle strength of hundreds of men and women, both when the pelvis was tilted and when it had been leveled with shims, and the increase in both strength and balance with a level pelvis is remarkable. By contrast, the relative weakness and diminished balance with an uncorrected pelvis leaves an athlete more vulnerable to injuries, in addition to the pain-causing effects of the resulting postural distortion.

Then, too, consider the effects of other postural distortions. Although the examples are almost limitless, take the case of a football player who has to turn to the left to block or to catch the football but whose pelvis is somewhat turned to the right by postural distortion. Every time he has to turn to the left, it's going to be more difficult for him, as he's turning against the "set" of his muscles, whereas turns to the right will be easy. By correcting the pelvic distortion, or by having the player work the opposite side of the field until the distortion is corrected, the player's performance can be enhanced. Simply put, in any sport where strength and balance are essential to championship performance, this kind of postural evaluation and correction can give top performers a critical edge in competition.

A Word to Employers

The cost to employers of posturally induced pain is staggering. From employee absenteeism and missed deadlines to higher employee health insurance rates and expensive pain-induced errors in job performance, the economic price of pain burdens employers and makes it harder for them to compete. It would be easy and inexpensive to establish a corporate postural screening program as a wellness benefit, as well as to provide incentives to employees who successfully complete training in postural balancing.

A Word to Parents

Wouldn't it be great to have your children screened for skeletal asymmetries early on so that they could be leveled up and spared years of pain and discomfort? In one fascinating study, "1.3–1.9 cm (1/2–3/4 in) leg length discrepancies in children between 1 1/2 and 15 years of age were outgrown (disappeared) in 7 of 11 children when leg length was equalized with a heel correction for 3–7 months."[1] Although further research is needed and not all children experienced the equalization, wouldn't it be wonderful to at least have that opportunity for your child to try? If parents will start asking to have their children posturally evaluated—even though it may take a while for some in the medical community to warm up to the idea—the increasing demand can eventually help to make postural evaluation a standard part of a physical examination.

A Word to Educators and Teachers

In our schools today, physical education emphasizes sports, which is all well and good, but children are missing out on an important part of true physical education. The majority of students will not grow up to play most of those sports on a regular basis, but every single student will grow up with a physical body to care for (or neglect). Wouldn't it be wise to give them training early on in the basics of postural balancing, thereby enabling them to maintain their physical bodies in good posture and avoid a lifetime of unnecessary musculoskeletal pain, medical problems, and healthcare expenses? We should change the physical education curricula to include training in such activities as daily stretching, structural balancing through resistance training and stretching, and the importance of good posture in maintaining good health and quality of life. That would be true "physical education."

A Word to Insurance Companies

In our society, the financial cost of musculoskeletal pain and its care is staggering, and the resulting rise in healthcare costs and medical insurance premiums is leading to calls for government controls on the health insurance industry. By covering the minimal cost involved in detecting and correcting skeletal asymmetries and perhaps offering health premium discounts for insureds who successfully complete training in postural balancing, health insurance companies could save themselves millions of dollars each year in payments for medical claims for pain diagnosis and treatment, and demonstrate that they are taking an active role in encouraging and supporting preventive healthcare, thereby possibly help to prevent the dreadful prospect of government regulation and management of health insurance.

A Word to Shoe Manufacturers

Shoes can be constructed so as to make it possible to easily add full foot sole corrections for skeletal asymmetries. The first manufacturers to do so will have a major sales feature to advertise and will reap the financial rewards accordingly. In addition, footwear of all types—dress, sport, casual, boots, sandals, slippers—can and should be offered that are absolutely level from heel to toe (no heel elevation). This would help the wearers reduce the tension (and consequent pain) in their legs, back, and neck caused by wearing elevated heels.

A Word to the Military, Police, and Firefighters

For the military, police, and firefighters, all of whose lives depend on top physical performance, as do the lives of those they protect, physical strength, balance, and the ability to perform their jobs without limitation from pain are mission-critical. Postural screening, especially for structural asymmetries, should be made a routine part of the hiring process, and members of those professions should be encouraged to keep themselves in postural balance for peak performance while on active duty.

A Word to Federal and State Governments

The many layers of government in this country and around the world spend billions of dollars each year in health-related programs. Wouldn't it make sense to save a significant portion of the billions in healthcare dollars currently spent for pain-related treatment by encouraging postural/skeletal evaluation by physicians and corrective training classes for patients so that people could learn how to reduce or eliminate their own musculoskeletal pain without expensive medical intervention?

A Word to Physicians

Physicians are in the perfect position to spearhead this effort, although for some it may require looking at this subject with new eyes. If the "official" medical approach says that small leg length and hemipelvis differences aren't significant and needn't be corrected, it may take a few open-minded physicians experimenting with making a brief skeletal asymmetry screening part of their new patient intake procedures in order to demonstrate the value and importance of correcting those small differences. For those physicians who focus on maintaining patient wellness, having staff members trained to do a detailed postural analysis and to provide advice on techniques for postural correction could greatly aid their efforts to help their patients keep themselves pain-free.

A Final Word to All Readers

If you found out that someone you knew had learned of a way to reduce or even eliminate your pain but hadn't told you about it, how would you feel? You get my point. If this approach makes sense to you, if it helps you control or eliminate your pain, don't keep it a secret. Spread the word. Tell others about it. Let them know that a lot of pain can be reduced, eliminated, or even prevented in the first place, and that they may be able to take control of much, if not all, of their musculoskeletal pain.

Although the basic postural analysis explained in this book will get you started on the right track, it's good to have your results confirmed by a properly trained professional if you can (more on that shortly). Ask to be posturally evaluated in more detail and have your children or other family members in your care evaluated as well. Encourage your friends and relatives to do the same. As an example, scoliosis screening of children is now routine in many schools across the country, and it would take less than a minute extra per student for a properly trained professional to perform a quick check for significant anatomical leg length or pelvic inequality. Although it may take a while for healthcare practitioners to start to adopt this type of postural screening and correction, your asking, combined with similar requests from thousands of others, can help to get these changes made. In the meantime, if you just keep monitoring your posture and working on your pain relief using the basic techniques outlined in this book, you'll do fine on your own.

Remember, though, what I said earlier: If a healthcare professional or any postural evaluator tells you that your skeletal asymmetry or postural distortion isn't significant, *only you, and you alone*, can ultimately decide whether that statement is true. Although a trained evaluator can give you excellent information about your posture and how to correct it, only you live in that body and know how it feels. For example, if putting a 1/8-inch lift under one foot relieves your pain and makes you feel better, it doesn't matter how "insignificant" anybody else thinks it is; it's significant to you, and you're in charge of your own healthcare and pain relief.

Although many readers will find the techniques presented in this book sufficient for their needs, others may be interested in learning this system in greater detail, whether for personal or professional use. If you're a member of one of the groups addressed earlier in this chapter—a healthcare provider, a coach or athlete, an employer, a parent, an educator, or just someone interested in learning how to use this system so that you can better monitor your own (and/or your family's) posture in order to achieve pain relief and better health, you can turn to the Appendix for more information on training seminars tailored to your needs.

Please help. Although this approach is not a "magic bullet" that will resolve all musculoskeletal pain, it will, if correctly and faithfully used, help to resolve a great deal of that pain and bring relief and comfort to so many of those who now suffer such pain needlessly. First, try this system for yourself, giving it time to work, and enjoy the relief from pain that it brings, along with the sense of wellness and empowerment as you realize that you now have control over your own musculoskeletal pain. Then, to end where we began in the Preface, "All I ask in return is that you share in this work by spreading the word to others that *a lot of pain is optional*, and that there *is* a way out. Once you know, it is important for you to help others to know."

"Freely ye have received, freely give."

Epilogue

I realize that some of the ideas I have presented may be in certain respects at variance with those commonly accepted by some in the various healing and/or fitness professions, but I have not written this book to be controversial. Rather, I have offered these ideas and techniques because I have seen them verified time and again, day after day, in my clinical practice, many times with clients who had exhausted all other pain relief options. I wanted to make this information more widely available to the millions who suffer needlessly with musculoskeletal pain, in the hope that by doing so I might help them to find relief. I can state my intentions no better than by quoting the powerful words of O. Otto Moore, former Chief Justice of the Colorado Supreme Court, in a dissenting opinion:

> *...perhaps my dissenting views are without merit. Nevertheless I have been required by conscience to set them forth for the single reason that although, admittedly, I may be wrong, I am not in doubt.*

And I am *not* in doubt.

I sincerely wish you and yours every blessing
of *Pain Relief for Life*.

Notes

Chapter 1

[1] Lehmkuhl, L. Don and Smith, Laura K. *Brunnstrom's Clinical Kinesiology* (4th Ed.). Philadelphia: F.A. Davis Company, 1983 (p. 50).

Chapter 1

[1] Specht DL, De Boer KF. "Anatomical leg length inequality, scoliosis and lordotic curve in unselected clinic patients." *Journal of Manipulative and Physiological Therapeutics,* July 1991, 14(6): 368–375.

[2] Travell, Janet G., M.D. and Simons, David G., M.D. *Myofascial Pain and Dysfunction, The Trigger Point Manual (Vol. 1).* Baltimore: Williams & Wilkins, 1983 (p. 103).

[3] Ibid (p. 651).

Chapter 11

[1] Ibid (p. 109).

Chapter 17

[1] Ibid (p. 107).

Appendix

Although the techniques presented in this book are sufficient to enable you to create your own pain-relief program successfully, many people have expressed a desire to learn these techniques in greater depth and detail, both for professional and personal use, as well as to acquire greater proficiency and understanding in a supervised classroom setting. As a result, I have created training seminars that are tailored to meet the needs of a wide range of interested groups. Some of those groups include:

▶ **Healthcare Professionals**

To offer healthcare professionals and their staff members hands-on training in performing more detailed evaluations of this type in a clinical setting, to go more deeply into the rationale for the corrective programs, and to provide a wider choice of options for therapeutic correction.

▶ **Athletes, Coaches, Trainers, and Fitness Professionals**

To get hands-on training in performing more detailed evaluations of this type and to learn to incorporate muscular balance evaluations into training routines in order to optimize athletic performance and help prevent injuries.

▶ **The General Public**

For individuals who want to learn this system of pain relief in a hands-on setting in order to keep themselves in optimum physical condition and to help reduce, eliminate, or prevent pain. Also for parents who want to learn this system in greater detail in order to be better able to evaluate and monitor their children's posture and eliminate postural problems early on.

▶ **Corporate Wellness Programs**

To give employees hands-on training in postural evaluation and self-correction for pain relief and to encourage personal responsibility and enthusiasm for wellness, thereby helping to reduce the employer's cost burden due to lost time, decreased productivity, and increased healthcare insurance premiums resulting from postural pain and injury.

▶ **Government Agencies, Including Police, Fire, and Military Units**

To provide supervisory and hiring staff members with hands-on training in postural screening and correction with this system, particularly for structural asymmetries, in order to ensure that front line personnel can perform their vital functions with optimum strength and balance, and without restriction due to postural pain.

Upon request, seminars can also be designed to meet the requirements of other groups.

For further information on these training seminars, please visit the *Pain Relief for Life* Website: *www.painreliefforlife.com*

Glossary

Anterior: Nearer to the front of the body.

Dorsiflexion: Bending of the ankle so that the toes move toward the knee.

Eversion: Movement of the foot at the ankle such that the sole of the foot moves outward.

Inferior: Further from the head or toward the lower part of a structure.

Inversion: Movement of the foot at the ankle such that the sole of the foot moves inward.

Lateral: Farther from the midline of the body or of a structure.

Medial: Closer to the midline of the body or of a structure.

Orthotics: Any devices added to the body that help to stabilize or protect a body part or improve function; in this book, orthotics is used to refer to arch supports for the feet (also called *orthoses*).

Plantar: Referring to the sole of the foot.

Plantar flexion: Bending of the ankle so that the toes move away from the knee.

Posterior: Nearer to the back of the body.

Pronation: A movement of the forearm that results in the palm of the hand facing inferiorly or posteriorly. Sometimes used to mean eversion of the foot, as when the medial longitudinal arch of the foot has collapsed.

Superior: Closer to the head or toward the upper part of a
                   structure.

Supination: A movement of the forearm that results in the palm of
                   the hand facing superiorly or anteriorly. Sometimes
                   used to mean inversion of the foot, as when the medial
                   longitudinal arch of the foot is high.

Bibliography

Aaberg, Everett. *Bio-Mechanically Correct.* Dallas: Realistic Individualized Professional Training Services, 1996.

Anderson, Bob. *Stretching.* Bolinas, Calif.: Shelter Publications, Inc., 1992.

Barker, Victor, M.D. *Posture Makes Perfect.* New York: Japan Publications, 1993.

Calais-Germain, Blandine. *Anatomy of Movement.* Seattle: Eastland Press, 1993.

Clemente, Carmine (Ed.). *Anatomy: A Regional Atlas of the Human Body (3rd Ed.).* Baltimore: Urban & Schwarzenburg, Inc., 1987.

Kendall, F. P., McCreary, E. K., Provance, P. G. *Muscles, Testing and Function, 4th Ed.* Baltimore: Williams & Wilkins, 1993.

Lehmkuhl, L. Don and Smith, Laura K. *Brunnstrom's Clinical Kinesiology* (4th Ed.). Philadelphia: F.A. Davis Company, 1983.

Taber's Cyclopedic Medical Dictionary, 17th Ed. Philadelphia: F.A. Davis Company, 1993.

Travell, Janet G., M.D. and Simons, David G., M.D. *Myofascial Pain and Dysfunction, The Trigger Point Manual.* Baltimore: Williams & Wilkins, 1983 (Vol. 1) and 1992 (Vol. 2).

Index

About the Author

AL SKROBISCH, C.N.M.T., B.A. is a neuromuscular therapist in private practice, specializing in pain relief. An enthusiastic and popular teacher and speaker, he has taught dozens of neuromuscular therapy seminars across the United States and Canada and is now introducing new seminars to teach this pain relief system.